AF260576

Table of Contents

Preface

Hi, I'm Rita, a health and fitness coach specializing in bespoke programs for unique individuals. I have spent years developing my skills, studying for my diploma in special population health and wellness needs, and educating myself in a myriad of exercise, nutrition and rehabilitation protocols. My joy in life is to help people be the best that they can be, as I understand what it is to be at rock bottom with no obvious way out. Whether it be excessive weight, mental fatigue, long covid, physical injury or something else entirely,we have all suffered set backs in our lives. But it is not what you have done in the past that matters, it is what you do next that is the measure of who you are. The fact that you have picked up this book means that you are ready to face your challenge head on, and I am proud of you for taking that first step.

I believe that there are three keys to health and recovery: fitness, nutrition, and mental well-being; and only when we bring these three together can we truly create a balanced life. I decided to study COVID-19 rehabilitation during the pandemic and learned as much as I could about how this savage disease affects people. The disease is not fair; it is random in who it hits, and I desire to help all individuals who were struck down in their prime to get back to their daily lives.

COVID-19 causes a lot of trauma, especially for patients with severe symptoms of the disease. After experiencing such a hard time in the hospital, and more so, in the ICU, the best one needs is to just heal completely and move on with their life.

However, this is usually not the case with COVID-19 patients that survive hospitalization. The disease may have physical, emotional, and psychological effects that affect patients well after the main symptoms have disappeared.

For more information, please visit my website www.thehealthandfitnesscoach.co.uk. or www.thehealthandfitnesscoach.com.

If any medical issues arise, be sure to contact your local health care professional and get relevant help as soon as possible.

Introduction

COVID-19 is an acronym where COVID represents coronavirus disease, and 19 denotes that the disease was identified in 2019. COVID-19 is caused by a type of coronavirus that is specifically known as the severe acute respiratory syndrome coronavirus 2 (SARS-CoV-2). The first cases of COVID-19 were reported in Wuhan, a city in Hubei province, in China. Due to the fact that the disease is highly contagious, it quickly spread within China, causing a lot of deaths and alarm. At that time, the disease was simply identified as a respiratory infection due to the symptoms that were exhibited by victims of the disease. Much panic took place in China, while for many other countries, it was still a story from a distant land.

On 31 December 2019, the first report of coronavirus disease was filed with the World Health Organization (WHO). However, there were no restrictions made at that time concerning movements, so the disease began to spread between countries as people continued to visit international tourist attractions, conferences, business meetings, and even religious ceremonies. There were not yet valid experiments that clearly highlighted how the disease spread from one individual to another, making the situation worse. The increase in COVID-19 cases in various countries triggered the WHO to declare the disease as a public health emergency at a global level on 30 January 2020. Although the whole world was in a state of emergency, the reality of it hadn't sunk into the minds of many. At least not until many people began to lose their loved ones to the disease in an abrupt manner.

Many hospitals around the world didn't have the relevant equipment to deal with the disease, so many people went to the hospitals but still perished. Due to the exponential rise in COVID-19 cases, patients outnumbered the equipment that was available, so even more families lost their loved ones every day.

No greater evidence was needed to declare that the world was faced with a pandemic. The WHO appropriately responded by declaring COVID-19 a global pandemic on 11 March 2020, after its cases were reported in 113 countries by that time (Khanna et al., 2020). This became the first pandemic declared by the WHO in almost a decade. The last declared global pandemic was the H1N1 in 2009.

The History of COVID-19

There are different types of coronaviruses. However, all of them are known to cause upper respiratory tract diseases whose symptoms can range from mild, like common colds, to severe, like pneumonia. Due to COVID-19, most people are now aware of coronaviruses that affect people, but there are others that affect cats, camels, and bats. It is reported that even those that affect animals can also evolve and affect human beings (National Foundation of Infectious Diseases, 2020). In animals, coronaviruses can cause diarrhea in pigs and cattle, hepatitis in mice, and upper respiratory infections in chickens.

The term 'coronaviruses' was coined due to the crown-like spikes that are found on the surface of coronaviruses. Corona is a Latin word for crown. It is believed that hundreds of coronaviruses exist, but by the year 2020, only 45 were officially recognized. Among the recognized ones, seven are known to cause illnesses in human beings, with four being characterized by severe symptoms. The coronavirus that causes COVID-19 is among the four that cause serious illnesses (National Institute of Allergy and Infectious Diseases, 2020).

In 2002, there was an epidemic caused by SARS-CoV, which led to the loss of about 774 lives throughout the world (NHS Choices, 2019). It is reported that this coronavirus was also first reported in China. The SARS-CoV-2 that causes COVID-19 is slightly different from the one that caused the 2002 epidemic. It is even more dangerous in that it can spread at a faster rate between symptomatic and asymptomatic individuals. Moreover, its symptoms can be extremely severe to the point of depriving its victims of breath.

The specific origins of the coronavirus 2 are not known. However, since the virus first emerged at a poultry and seafood market in Wuhan, China, some assume that it might have been transmitted from animals to humans.

Coronaviruses, like any other viruses, multiply themselves when they are in their hosts. However, there can be some mistakes that happen during the replication process. If these mistakes are incorporated into the nucleic acid of the virus, new forms may result. It is important that people follow the guidelines for staying safe from the virus at all times.

Stronger Than Warriors?

The size of SARS-CoV-2 ranges between 50 and 200 nanometers—so small, yet it has turned the whole world upside-down (Varga et al., 2020). COVID-19 has instilled fear, depression, and anxiety, even in the most courageous people in this world. As of 1 May 2021, over 3 million people have succumbed to COVID-19 throughout the globe, both the young and the old (WorldOMeter, 2020).

After COVID-19 was declared a global pandemic by the WHO, many countries slipped into national lockdowns to restrict movements. These lockdowns minimized the spread of the coronavirus 2 at the expense of economic growth, international business opportunities, and freedom of movement for citizens of different countries. Some people even lost their livelihood as they could not go on with the business that hinged on their survival and that of their families. Some children lost the opportunity for education as their parents could not afford to pay their fees any longer. Thousands of people lost their jobs as companies halted their everyday business due to the pandemic. Online businesses became the order of the day, and services that could not be offered online were greatly affected.

Even after lockdown restrictions were eased, people are still scared of being the next victim of the virus. All people are now making efforts to observe high levels of hygiene—all because of the coronavirus. Everywhere, people have their masks on. Sanitizing and regular hand washing have become the norm. You cannot enter the shops, salons, hospitals, schools, and various workplaces without a mask and sanitizing your hands.

You Can Survive

Although there are many rehabilitation programs for people who survived other illnesses, COVID-19 is relatively new, and therefore there are no stipulated rehabilitation procedures. However, we are aware that COVID patients are affected by the disease to varying extents. They could be mild or severe, to the extent of requiring hospitalization or being put in the ICU. It has been reported that in the United Kingdom, 50% of patients that are hospitalized due to COVID-19 may need continuous care to improve the long-term effects of the disease (Ayoubkhani et al., 2021). For example, the efficacy of their upper respiratory system may become highly compromised. Whichever the case might be, you can survive.

Apart from physical well-being, COVID-19 affects the mental stability of many people. Most survivors of the disease are left with a constellation of negative emotions such as stress, anxiety, fear, depression, and loss of self-worth. They can't believe they were on the verge of leaving their families and friends just like that. If you are one of such people, this book will help you to fight back and take back your life. It will guide you toward recovering your health, releasing negative emotions, rebuilding hope for the future, and making strides to your destiny with bravery.

Chapter 1: Symptoms of COVID-19

People who contract the coronavirus exhibit a wide range of symptoms, from mild to severe ones. Symptoms among individuals may be influenced by factors such as age, living conditions, socioeconomic status, and other factors that we will discuss in this chapter. This chapter will explore the various symptoms of COVID-19, together with other aspects connected to them.

Overall Symptoms

In some people, the coronavirus may not cause any symptoms at all. For those that show symptoms of COVID-19, the effect can be short or long term, depending on how long they can persist. It is also important to note that it may take between 2 days and 2 weeks before symptoms may show in a person with COVID-19.

Primary Symptoms

Not all symptoms that have been reported for COVID-19 have the same severity. Moreover, some are more common than others. In this section, the focus will be on the symptoms of COVID-19 that are common among patients.

1. Shortness of Breath

One of the severe symptoms of COVID-19 is shortness of breath, which is clinically known as dyspnea. This is a situation where the COVID patient begins to gasp for oxygen, as though there is no more oxygen in the air. They begin to feel unable to provide their lungs with the oxygen that they need. Simply said, the shortness of breath that is caused by COVID-19 makes it difficult for one to breathe deeply, leaving them with no option for survival other than to make shallow, more frequent breaths. For those that had the experience of this symptom and survived, they liken the scenario to "drowning with no water" (Giovinco, 2020).

COVID-related dyspnea is usually evident any time between days 4 and 10 after infection by the coronavirus 2 (Fraley, 2020). Shortness of breath takes place when the muscles in your lungs take much of the work that is required in breathing.

Normally, breathing should be a result of the combined effort by the lung muscles and the diaphragm. This usually takes place when you are relaxed. However, being relaxed is not an option, especially in severe cases of COVID-19. A lot of stress is involved, causing other effects such as a racing heart.

While there are other diseases that cause shortness of breath, doctors have found a way to distinguish between the shortness of breath that is caused by COVID-19 and that caused by other diseases. Other diseases that cause inadequacy of breath include heart disease, asthma, and chronic obstructive pulmonary disease (COPD). It has been determined that the shortness of breath that is caused by COVID-19 is characterized by instant drops in oxygen saturation after slight exertion. Oxygen saturation refers to the extent to which there is a balance in the number of red blood cells that are impregnated with oxygen.

Your next question might be, "How does COVID-19 cause shortness of breath?" Normally, oxygen should pass through the air sacs, into the capillaries of the lungs, before being distributed to all parts of the body. This normal movement of oxygen is disrupted in COVID-19 patients. When one contracts the coronavirus, the immune system is triggered against the virus. This causes white blood cells to release chemokine, which are inflammatory cells that play an important role in fighting pathogens. The activity of the chemokines results in SAR-CoV-2 cells being destroyed. The continuous fight between the coronavirus and the immune system results in the accumulation of pus, which is the resultant combination of excess fluid and dead cells in the lungs. The pus clogs the airways in the lungs, thereby distracting the undisturbed movement of oxygen. This situation in the lungs is exhibited by symptoms such as shortness of breath and coughing.

2. Fever

Fever is a condition where the body temperature rises to levels above normal, usually above 100 F. It is also known as pyrexia or hyperthermia. The body can respond to infection by raising its temperature as a way to fight the pathogens that would have invaded it. Therefore, a short-term fever can be helpful to an infected body. On the contrary, fever that persists for longer periods is a cause for concern and would require immediate attention by health professionals.

It is also crucial to note that although fever is regarded as one of the major symptoms of COVID-19, some patients with the disease may never experience it at all. In one study, an investigation on 213 participants that were diagnosed with mild coronavirus disease showed that only 11.6% of them confirmed fever to be one of the symptoms that they experienced (Kim et al., 2020). Fever alone cannot determine whether an individual has COVID-19 or not because there are other diseases that cause fever as well. For instance, infection by the influenza virus can also cause fever in human beings.

Let's explore the science behind having a fever. The temperature of your body is controlled by a part of the brain called the hypothalamus. When the hypothalamus alters the set point for your body temperature from its normal position moving upward, you might feel a little cold, even when everyone else around you feels fine. Your response to this chilling experience might be to wear warm clothes. If not, your body may start shivering to generate enough heat to counter the cold experience. This results in an elevated body temperature above the normal ranges.

3. Coughing

Coughing is a normal reflex action that involves vigorously expelling air from the lungs. It helps to remove any unwanted material that could have clogged the air passages in the lungs. Such irritants could be dust, mucus, or even pus, as is the case with COVID-19.

Coughs can be categorized based on their duration as follows:

- An **acute cough** does not exceed three weeks.
- A **subacute cough** might exceed three weeks but does not go beyond eight weeks.
- A **chronic** cough stretches beyond eight weeks.

The research that has been done so far shows that the cough that is caused by COVID-19 sticks around for an average of 19 days. This means that the COVID-19-related cough is classified as acute, but it gets more severe as time elapses. However, it has been reported that even after the period when one can transmit the coronavirus to others, COVID-19 survivors may experience a post-viral cough (World Health Organization, 2020a). The post-viral cough may be due to the damage to the lining of your airways as a result of the inflammatory response to infection by the coronavirus. It could also be due to increased sensitivity of the coughing reflex after infection by the coronavirus.

Another way of classifying coughs is by determining whether they are productive or dry.

A productive cough is accompanied by mucus, while a dry one is not. The cough that emanates from infection by COVID-19 is dry.

4. Fatigue

Fatigue refers to an overall state of exhaustion or tiredness. This term is often confused with drowsiness, but the two words describe different things. Feeling sleepy can be a symptom of fatigue, but on its own, it is not fatigue. COVID-19 can make you feel like your energy has been drained, hence making you feel tired and less vigorous in your daily activities.

Less Common Symptoms

Some symptoms of the coronavirus are less common among patients. This means that they may appear in some patients and not in others. The fact that these symptoms are designated as "less common" does not imply that they are less important or severe. Although they are less common, the symptoms that are highlighted in this section may become severe and may contribute to critical cases of COVID-19.

1. Headache

Headaches are also part of a group of symptoms that are related to coronavirus disease. However, the exact point along the progression of the disease during which headaches begin has not yet been determined. Available reports from COVID-19 patients show that some experienced headaches during the onset of the disease while others experienced them late in the infection phase. People with migraines may experience headaches before other symptoms that are typical of COVID-19, like fever, are evident. Headaches are more common symptoms of coronavirus disease in people who are below the age of 65.

A report from the WHO showed that 13.6% of 55,000 cases experienced headaches (World Health Organization, 2020b). Similar results were reported by the Centers for Disease Control and Prevention (CDC) that revealed that the incidences of headaches among hospitalized patients ranged between 9.6% and 21.3% (Garg, 2020).

Headaches are a common health-related concern, even in people without COVID-19. This makes the ability to differentiate between COVID-related and any other headaches difficult, and this can be a daunting task because the headaches are more or less similar. However, here are some of the characteristics of a headache that is caused by COVID-19:

- It is bilateral, meaning it is felt on both sides of the head.
- Its intensity is usually moderate to severe, rarely light.
- It generates a pulsing sensation in the head.
- Bending over may make it feel worse.

To further differentiate between COVID headaches and migraine headaches, there are two major factors to consider:

- COVID-related headaches are not coupled with symptoms such as sensitivity to sound and light, as is the case with migraines.
- If you have a headache and feel feverish at the same time, the headache is more likely to be COVID-related than migraine-related. Fevers are common in viral infections but not in migraines.

2. Sensory Debility

COVID-19 may also affect the senses of taste and smell. This is a common symptom of respiratory tract infections, including influenza. The sense of taste is closely related to that of smell; therefore, any malfunction in one may affect the other. In fact, in approximately 95% of the cases where there is a loss of taste, a loss of smell is also evident (Selad-Schulman, 2020a). This is usually the case with COVID-19. In COVID patients, the loss of smell and taste may also be coupled with a dry nose, which is neither runny nor stuffy.

Loss of taste or smell can occur at the onset of infection or later on. There are many cases when COVID-related loss of smell and taste were reported to happen before other symptoms of the disease (Samaranayake et al., 2020). However, another study highlighted that loss of smell in COVID patients was more frequently noted in outpatients than admitted patients (Yan et al., 2020). This could imply that loss of smell is a symptom that occurs before the other adverse symptoms that require admission to the hospital. Alternatively, it could mean that COVID patients may lose their sense of smell, even after recovering from the other symptoms, in which case the loss of smell would have taken place at a later stage of the progression of the disease.

Loss of taste and smell that emanates from infection by the SARS-CoV-2 tends to last for longer periods, unlike in infections caused by other viruses. On average, loss of smell and taste may continue for about 8 days but can stretch up to 28 days (Klopfeinstein et al., 2020; Seladi-Schulman, 2020a)

Let's briefly discuss the science behind the loss of taste and smell in COVID-19 patients. Sudden loss of smell is referred to as anosmia. Studies have revealed that the SARS-CoV-2 requires angiotensin-converting enzyme 2 (ACE2) and a protease called transmembrane protease serine type 2 (TMPRSS2) as receptors for it to gain entry into human cells. Therefore, the virus can only attack cells that express these proteins. Although there are different types of cells that express these proteins, such cells are abundant in the throat, nose, and upper bronchial pathways. In the nose, the expression of the ACE2 and TMPRSS2 is evident in the respiratory epithelium (RE) and olfactory sensory epithelium (OSE). The cells in these epitheliums, especially the OSE, are responsible for keeping the sensory neurons and mucus layer in good health so that neurons are properly activated by smells. When the epithelium cells are invaded by the SARS-CoV-2, they are unable to perform their function properly, and so odors cannot properly activate the neuron. This results in reduced or complete loss of smell (Kay, 2020).

Not much information is available to explain the loss of taste in COVID patients. However, it is assumed that since the senses of taste and smell are highly related, the loss of taste might be a result of the loss of smell.

To find out if you have lost your sense of smell, you can try smelling things that have characteristically strong smells, like fresh garlic or coffee beans. You can also determine the inactivity of your sense of taste by eating foods with different tastes and figure out if your sense of taste is able to pick those tastes. For example, you can try pretzels for saltiness, chocolates for sweetness, coffee for bitterness, and citrus for sourness.

2. Sore Throat

In other illnesses such as colds, sore throat is often experienced at the onset of infection. The most probable explanation for this is that viruses that cause respiratory diseases are usually inhaled through the mouth. As they move through the respiratory tract, they might begin to replicate in the cells on the throat, causing soreness. This uncomfortable pain in the throat is also one of the symptoms of COVID-19. However, with coronavirus disease, it is currently unclear at what point during the progression of the disease that the throat may become sore.

The reports from various studies show that a sore throat is not a common symptom of COVID-19. Two studies with relatively small numbers of participants reported 5% (Lima, 2020) and 7.1% (Su et al., 2020) cases of COVID-related sore throat in their results. In a larger study that involved 55,000 confirmed cases of COVID-19, 13.9% experienced sore throat as one of their symptoms (World Health Organization, 2020a).

3. Gastrointestinal Disturbances

People with COVID-19 may experience gastrointestinal challenges. These symptoms are either accompanied by other respiratory symptoms or occur alone. The most common gastrointestinal complications with regard to COVID are diarrhea, vomiting, and nausea. Since COVID-19 symptoms widely vary among individuals, gastrointestinal symptoms also vary among populations.

- Some people **lose their appetite** after contracting COVID-19. This symptom usually occurs together with other gastrointestinal symptoms. Sometimes, the loss of appetite may be due to the loss of smell and taste, which might rob COVID patients of the joy associated with eating.

- In one study that focused on the digestive symptoms that occurred in patients with mild COVID cases, it could be concluded **diarrhea** coupled with respiratory symptoms is a common symptom of COVID (Han et al., 2020). Among the 206 COVID-19 patients that participated in the study, 69 of them had a combination of respiratory and gastrointestinal symptoms, while 48 only had diarrhea. The overall occurrence of diarrhea in the patient, according to this study, was 56.8%.

- People suffering from COVID-19 may also find it difficult to hold the food that they eat in their stomachs; once they eat, they **vomit**. This symptom is more common in children that are infected by the coronavirus than in adults. In a review that was done by Yuan Tian and colleagues, they reported an approximate maximum of 15.9% of vomiting cases in adults with COVID-19, against the 66.7% that was recorded for infected children (Tian et al., 2020).

- COVID-19 patients may also experience nausea, gastrointestinal bleeding, and abdominal pain.

As explained before, the SARS-CoV-2 gains entrance into cells through the ACE2 receptors. It is also suggested that the virus uses the same route in attacking the digestive system. In fact, the availability of ACE2 receptors in the digestive tract is 100 times more than it is in the respiratory tract (Yetman, 2020a). Therefore, the likelihood that the coronavirus can affect the gastrointestinal tract and cause symptoms such as diarrhea and vomiting is high.

Concerns have been raised with regard to the fact that people with gastrointestinal disorders might be at a higher risk of contracting COVID-19. However, there is no research that supports that notion at the moment. Therefore, according to the information that is currently available, people with conditions such as inflammatory bowel disease (IBD) have the same risk of contracting COVID-19 as those that do not have the condition.

4. Muscle Pain

In the field of medicine, muscle pain is known as myalgia. This symptom is common for viral infections. Like any other virus, SARS-CoV-2 can trigger inflammation of the tissues of muscles. The coronavirus also damages muscle fibers, thereby causing muscle pain. When your body is infected by the coronavirus, it responds by initiating an inflammatory response, and this can cause abnormal tissue breakdown. This may also contribute to the pain that COVID patients experience in their muscles.

The muscle pain that is caused by coronavirus infection is not the same as that of workouts in that it is more generalized. Pain that is caused by exercise is usually specific to certain muscles that would have been stretched during the workout. You can also differentiate muscle pain caused by the coronavirus by considering the time taken for the pain to resolve. Muscle pain from exercise takes less time to resolve—usually between 48 and 72 hours. In contrast, the pain caused by a viral infection can stretch up to several weeks or even months after the body is free from infection. The muscle pain that emanates from coronavirus infection may be felt during movements such as walking or when you actually touch the muscles.

5. Shaking With Chills

Chills, which are periods of intense shivering that are coupled with feeling cold, and sometimes paleness, have been reported in COVID patients. They are usually associated with fever, or they can reflect the beginning of feverish symptoms. This implies that chills are not a direct indication that one has contracted COVID-19 since they can result from infection by any other virus other than the coronavirus. However, they are listed among the symptoms of COVID-19 because, in conjunction with other symptoms, they may help to determine the likelihood that the sickness that one might be suffering from is COVID-19 or not.

When you get infected with a virus like coronavirus, the inflammatory response triggers a raise in temperature in a bid to get rid of the infection at a faster rate. The chills and shivering help your body to generate more heat and raise the body temperature. This is the reason why chills may reduce or stop when the body temperature is above normal and you have a fever. It is clear that chills are mainly associated with fever, which is one of the common symptoms of COVID-19 infection.

Sometimes, chills may become intense, causing tremors. In this case, the whole body shakes, not just some parts of the body. In one study that involved 24,410 COVID patients, 11.6% of them reported that they experienced these severe chills (Grant et al., 2020).

It is difficult to determine whether the chills that you might be experiencing are COVID-related or not without a COVID test. However, if the chills are accompanied by fever, muscle pain, headache, shivering, and other symptoms that we described in this chapter, then there might be a probability that you have COVID-19. It is misleading to consider only chills in determining whether you have COVID.

6. Pink Eye

The coronavirus may also affect the eyes and cause conjunctivitis, which is also called pink eye. It is assumed that an average of 2% of people that have COVID-19 will get coronavirus-related conjunctivitis (Mukamal, 2020). COVID-related conjunctivitis happens when the SARS-CoV-2 infects the conjunctiva, the part of the eye that covers the inner side of the eyelids as well as the white part of the eye. You might have pink eye if your eyes are red, swollen, and itchy. Assuming that you have COVID-19 just by considering conjunctivitis is misleading because other bacteria and viruses can infect the conjunctiva and exhibit similar symptoms. However, considering other symptoms that emanate from infection with the coronavirus can be helpful in providing a more accurate assumption.

The virus that causes COVID-19 is usually transmitted through coughing and sneezing by an infected individual. One can also contract the virus by getting into contact with infected surfaces prior to touching their eyes, nose, or mouth. This implies that SARS-CoV-2 can also be transmitted through the eyes. As I highlighted before, the coronavirus that causes COVID-19 enters human cells by tricking the cells into assuming that it is the ACE2 enzyme. It, therefore, uses the ACE2 receptors to gain entrance into the cells. ACE2 receptors have been identified on the retina of the human eye, thereby making it an easy target by the virus. When the virus successfully affects the eye, it causes the eye to be red.

7. Stuffy or Runny Nose

Reports from the WHO show that a stuffy or runny nose is one of the symptoms of COVID-19, though it is less common than the other symptoms such as fever, fatigue, and dry cough. A stuffy or runny nose is a result of nasal congestion, which makes breathing through the nose difficult and uncomfortable. You feel like your nose is blocked, so inhaled and exhaled air can't pass freely. Like many other symptoms that are linked to COVID-19, a stuffy or runny nose cannot be used to give a final decision as to whether one is infected with COVID-19 or not. This is especially true during the time of the year when allergies and influenza are more prevalent.

You could consider the other symptoms that you are experiencing, if any. They could help to narrow down the possibilities of infection. Another factor that you could look at if you are suspecting that the stuffy or runny nose that you are experiencing could be a reflection that you have COVID-19 is your lifestyle. Have you been wearing a mask in public, properly washing your hands with running water and soap, sanitizing your hands, and keeping social distance? If your answer is 'no,' then you have every reason to be concerned, and a COVID test is necessary.

8. Rash

COVID-19 patients may also have rashes that may or may not occur together with other symptoms. There are various types of rashes that exist with regard to COVID-19, and these include:

- **COVID toes and fingers**: Also known as chilblains, this type of rash refers to purplish and reddish bumps that occur on the fingers or toes and is common in younger people. Chilblains are more COVID-related than they could be with any other disease.
- **Oral rash**: This type of rash causes the lips to be sore, dry, and scaly. Sometimes, the soreness can extend to the inside of the mouth.

- **The hive-type**: This type of rash is also known as the urticaria. These are itchy, raised bumps that occur on the skin. They can appear and disappear within hours. The hive-type rash usually begins with pain in the soles or palms but can appear on any part of the skin. This type of rash causes the lips and eyelids to swell. Most of the patients that have hive-type rashes report their appearance at the onset of their infection by the coronavirus. However, it can persist even long after the infection is gone.

- **Eczema on the exposed chest and neck**: This rash can appear on anyone, regardless of whether they have a history of dermatological conditions or not. It appears on the neck and part of the chest that is exposed to sunlight rays. Eczema can persist for elongated periods of time.

- **The "prickly heat" type**: This rash is also referred to as the erythematous vesicular rash or erythematous papular rash. It can appear on any part of the body, though it is commonly witnessed on the elbows and knees. It also appears on the feet and back of hands. The prickly heat rash can remain on the skin for days, even up to weeks.

Who Is Affected by COVID?

There are no exceptions as to who can contract COVID-19. However, there are differences in severity of symptoms among individuals. These discrepancies are due to various factors that make other people more vulnerable to the effects of infection by the SARS-CoV-2. This implies that even when two individuals contract the coronavirus, the symptoms that they might show are different. At the same time, even if they would show the same symptoms, the severity of the symptoms is never the same. Therefore, this section explores the different groups of people that are most affected by the coronavirus. To effectively address this, we will discuss the factors that affect the severity of COVID-19 symptoms. Some of such factors are:

1. Age

The severity of COVID-19 symptoms increases with age. This means that the older you are, the greater the probability that you will fall seriously ill if you contract coronavirus disease. People who are over 85 have the highest risk of exhibiting coronavirus symptoms in their most severe form.

One of the reasons why this happens is that the immune system becomes weaker and more compromised as one gets older. A weaker immune system makes it easier for the coronavirus to attack the cells with less resistance from the body. Another reason is that the lung tissue hardens as one ages. As a result, those who are older find it difficult to heal after a SARS-CoV-2 infection. Older people also have a higher risk of inflammation. This causes organ damage that can become worse if they contract coronavirus disease. Lastly, conditions such as type 2 diabetes and high blood pressure are more prevalent in older members of society. These chronic conditions make them more susceptible to infection with the coronavirus.

2. Other Chronic Conditions

People who have other chronic conditions are at a higher risk of getting seriously sick due to COVID-19. This includes people who might be young but have other underlying conditions that might make them more prone to contracting the more severe form of the disease. These chronic illnesses include the following:

- **Heart disease**: COVID-19 mostly affects the respiratory system, especially the air pathways and lungs. However, it also has effects on the circulatory system, particularly the heart, because this organ works hand in hand with the lungs in transporting oxygen to all parts of the body. When the lungs are incapacitated, as is the case in people with COVID-19, then the heart has to work a lot harder to ensure that all tissues still receive the required amount of oxygen while removing the carbon dioxide. Therefore, people who already have heart disease as an underlying condition may suffer more severe symptoms due to the disease. Simply said, COVID-19 may worsen their health condition by escalating heart disease. Types of heart disease to look out for include pulmonary hypertension, coronary artery disease, congenital heart disease, and cardiomyopathy.

- **Diabetes**: Both diabetes types 1 and 2 are risk factors for coronavirus disease. Type 1 diabetes is found in people that do not produce insulin at all in their bodies. When an individual produces insulin, but their body does not respond to it, then the condition becomes known as type 2 diabetes. People with type 2 diabetes are also at risk of type 1 diabetes. However, both types of diabetes result in the accumulation of blood sugar. As a result, there are high concentrations of sugar in the blood. High blood sugar levels provide a conducive environment for viruses, including the coronaviruses, to thrive. This implies that people with diabetes make it easier for the SARS-CoV-2 to attack their cells and multiply. This increases the probability of experiencing a severe form of coronavirus disease. Additionally, type 1 and type 2 diabetes weaken the immune system and increase the chances of inflammation. A weaker immune system cannot effectively respond to infection by the coronavirus, thereby increasing the risk of infection, as well as the progression of the disease.

- **Lung disease**: Diseases that affect the airways and whole lungs present an increased risk of causing serious illness due to SARS-CoV-2 infection. Such conditions include asthma, pulmonary fibrosis, chronic obstructive pulmonary disease (COPD), and interstitial lung disease. Since these diseases cause inflammation and damage to the lungs, infection by COVID-19 will only worsen the situation that is already present.

- **Conditions that weaken the immune system**: All conditions that weaken the immune system increase the health risk that is posed by COVID-19 in individuals. Some of such conditions are HIV/AIDS, cancer treatments, organ transplants, chronic kidney disease, and bone marrow transplants. All these conditions compromise the efficiency of the immune system in fighting against viral infections, including the coronaviruses.

People with underlying conditions should connect themselves to doctors so that they get assistance immediately if the need arises. If they experience symptoms that might be associated with COVID-19, they should report them to a health professional with immediate effect. For conditions that require medication, patients should always have a supply and take their medication as recommended by health professionals. For example, diabetic individuals should appropriately take their medication to keep their blood sugar levels at low levels.

Long COVID Effects

Have you ever heard about long COVID? For you to understand what long COVID is, I will start by explaining the known developmental stages of COVID-19. Of course, there may be variation here and there in how COVID progresses in different individuals, but we are going to discuss the general timeline as far as the disease is concerned.

Progression of COVID-19

Here are the stages that determine the progression of COVID-19:

1. **Incubation**: After contracting the coronavirus, individuals do not show symptoms immediately, but they can spread the virus to others. Studies show that a person is more infectious about 48 hours before they begin to show symptoms of COVID-19 (Sakay, 2020). However, there should be a short timeframe that gives the virus the time to infect human cells and start causing damage. This stage can span up to 6 days after infection.

2. **Prodromal**: This marks the appearance of early symptoms of illness. Usually, the appearance of symptoms begins to appear during the first week. For some people, the symptoms appear gradually, while for some, they hit hard from the onset. Symptoms like diarrhea, fever, muscle pain, joint aches, and reduced taste and smell abilities are experienced any time between the 4th and 10th day after infection.

3. **Acute**: The more serious symptoms presented in the 'prodromal' section above begin to

increase in severity at this stage. COVID-19 begins to mature into a full-blown disease at this stage. This stage normally spans between day 10 and day 15 after infection. When a COVID patient reaches this stage, they need hospitalization, or more specifically, the ICU. If the infection is realized earlier, patients may never have to reach the acute stage because intervention will be done earlier.

4. **Convalescence**: The convalescence stage marks the period after day 14. In other words, COVID-19 should be full-blown in 2 weeks, after which the patients either begin to recover or become worse and die. Convalescence may span up to a week, that is, up to day 22 after infection. For those that recover, fever disappears within 72 hours before day 22 (Sakay, 2020). Transmission does not take place during recovery, although it is recommended that patients wait for at least 3 more days before they can start mingling with other people.

More serious symptoms such as pneumonia, shortness of breath, and coughing usually appear after the 7-day mark. At this point, some individuals can either have dry or wet coughs. A wet cough may contain mucus and lung cells that have been destroyed by the virus. These symptoms are more serious, and so they present the onset of the acute phase of progression of COVID-19.

Do I Have Long COVID?

Having looked at how COVID-19 progresses, let's discuss long COVID. The term "long COVID" refers to symptoms of COVID-19 that remain even after an individual has fully recovered from the disease. Basically, long COVID can be well described in two ways:

- COVID-19 symptoms that extend to periods between 4 and 12 weeks before disappearing.
- Symptoms that last beyond 12 weeks and have no other explanation except for COVID-19.

If any of these symptoms last for more than 4 weeks, you need to contact a health practitioner for appropriate assistance. Let them know exactly how and what you feel, and they will help you determine whether you are suffering from long COVID or not. Procrastinating a little longer might cause you to suffer more severe effects from long COVID.

Chapter 2: Phases and Treatments

In Chapter 1, I highlighted some of the stages that describe the progression of COVID-19. We are going to discuss COVID-19 progression in more detail in this chapter. In addition to exploring the different phases, we will also look at the treatments that are available for each phase. However, before delving in, let's look at how the SARS-CoV-2 can be contracted. How does it gain access to your body?

Transmission of the Virus

As long as you do not have direct contact with the droplets infected with the coronavirus 2, you are safe from COVID-19. Typically, individuals are exposed to infected droplets when others who have the virus sneeze or cough. That way, the virus in droplets falls directly onto the facial area, where they can enter the body through the eyes, nose, or mouth. Sometimes, hands act as aids for transmission also. For example, if you touch surfaces with infected droplets and touch body parts on your face afterward, you transfer the coronavirus-infected droplets into your body.

The way SARS-CoV-2 is transmitted is very direct and straightforward. This makes it relatively simple to prevent infection by this virus. Research has shown that COVID-19 is not an airborne disease because the droplets from sneezing, coughing, and speaking are too heavy to hang on in the air or travel long distances. As a result, they fall down onto surfaces. This implies that you can protect yourself from contracting the virus by keeping your distance from other people, approximately two meters. This is the essence of social distancing. Wearing your cloth face mask also shows that you care, not only for yourself but for others, too. In the event that you sneeze, cough, or speak, you neither infect surfaces that others will touch nor infect them directly.

Avoid touching surfaces because you do not know whether they are clean or not. You might get infected if you do. In the event that you touch surfaces, or you are not sure if you did, just make it a habit to disinfect your hands with an alcohol-based sanitizer. Such sanitizers have been proven to destroy all types of microorganisms, including bacteria and viruses. Most organizations have sanitizing facilities that you can access upon entering their premises.

Washing your hands with soap and under clean, running water is one of the prime ways to protect yourself against infection. It's not just a matter of washing your hands, but properly doing so. The CDC (2019) provided a general procedure for effectively washing your hands:

- **Use warm or cold running water to wet your hands prior to applying soap**. It is important to use running water because water from, say, a dish can be contaminated by the person that previously used it. In such a case, you might infect yourself instead. Using soap is more effective than washing your hands with water only. The surfactants in soaps assist in lifting the virus from your skin, making them less attached and easier to remove.

- **After adding soap to your wet hands, rub them together to create lather**. Be sure to lather every part of your hands—between your fingers, at the back of your hands, and under your nails. The process of lathering and scrubbing your hands helps to weaken the attachment of dirt, oils, and microorganisms from your skin.

- **Be sure to scrub your hands for at least 20 seconds**. Use a timer if need be, or you can just count from 1 to 20. To make it more fun, just hum the "Happy Birthday" song from beginning to end, two times. Longer washing periods correlate with the more efficient removal of dirt and germs.

- **Use clean, running water to rinse your hands**. Why not just leave the soap on the skin? Rinsing is basically done for two reasons. First, while soap lifts dirt from your skin, it doesn't wash it off, and you need water to do this. Second, soap may become irritating if it remains on the skin, so it is best to remove it with running water. Standing water is not recommended because it increases the chances of reinfection.

- **Air-dry your hands**. Studies show that it is easier for microorganisms to be transferred between wet hands than dry ones (Patrick et al., 1997). This is why drying your hands after washing them is of paramount importance. The CDC suggests that you can also use a clean towel to dry your hands, but you can never be too sure, especially in shared spaces. The towels may be somehow contaminated with the virus. On the other hand, you can never go wrong with air-drying.

Structure of the Coronavirus 2

To enhance a better understanding of the lifecycle of the coronavirus and the phases that COVID patients go through after infection, it is crucial to briefly explore the structure of the virus. We will, therefore, explore the structure of the virus with regard to how it infects human cells. The virus that causes COVID-19 has four major structural proteins that make it possible for the virus to infect human cells. Three of these proteins are glycoproteins, namely spike (S), envelope (E), and membrane (M) glycoproteins. The fourth protein is the nucleocapsid (N) protein. There are other accessory proteins that are important in the life cycle of the coronavirus 2.

The spike protein is found on the outside of the virus, where it protrudes from its surface. The virus uses spike proteins attached to human host cells before entering them. As I mentioned earlier, the coronavirus 2 attaches to the host cells by binding to the ACE2 receptors on the surface of these cells. The role of the spike proteins is made easier by furin-like protease in host cells. This protease cleaves the spike proteins into two parts—S1 and S2 subunits. The S1 part is the one that identifies the host range that the virus can infect. This subunit also identifies the cells that express the ACE2 receptor. The S2 part aids the attachment of the virus to the human cells, thereby initiating the infection process.

The nucleocapsid protein is bound to the virus's nucleic acid. Since it is closely associated with the RNA of the SARS-CoV-2, the nucleocapsid protein is highly involved in the multiplication of the virus. For the coronavirus to increase in numbers in the host cell, its nucleic acid should be replicated into many copies that will be used to assemble more viruses. When more copies of the virus are produced in the human host cell, they release viruses that go on to infect other healthy cells.

The shape of the envelope of the virus is determined by the membrane protein. This protein also stabilizes nucleocapsid proteins by binding to them. This process increases the efficiency of the viral assembly after the viral genome is expressed using the human cell machinery. The envelope protein is the smallest of all the main proteins of SARS-CoV-2. It is also involved in the production and maturation process of the coronavirus.

The Journey Through COVID-19

In the event that you do not observe the recommendations that have been described earlier in this chapter, the risk of contracting the virus that causes COVID-19 is elevated. Now, we are going to discuss the different changes that the virus causes to the body as COVID-19 progresses. The five stages that are going to be expounded are the virus in the nasal cavity, replication in the lungs and altered immune system, hypoxia and pneumonia, acute respiratory distress syndrome (ARDS), and recovery.

Virus in the Nasal Chambers

After one has been infected with the coronavirus through any of the means that we discussed earlier, the first part of the body where the virus usually establishes itself is the nasal passages. Infection in other parts of the body, such as the lungs, is usually an extension of the infection in the nasal cavity. This then implies that wearing masks does not only protect others, apart from the person wearing the mask. Face masks also help to protect the nose, and hence, the nasal passages from infection. If the nasal passages are well protected from being infected by the virus, then the first establishment of the virus in the human body is hindered.

The ACE2 receptor that the virus uses to gain entrance into the human cells is present in abundance in nasal lining cells. The surface of lower airway cells also contains the ACE2, but in fewer numbers as compared to the nasal lining. This explains why the nasal cavity is highly infected by SARS-CoV-2.

The infection of the cells in the nasal lining begins with the attachment of the spike protein of the virus to the ACE2 receptor of the nasal lining cells. It is important to note that the spike protein of the coronavirus 2 only forms strong bonds with the ACE2 receptors in human and bat cells. After the binding process between the spike proteins of the virus and the ACE2 receptors, the cell membranes of the virus and the host cell fuse together.

The surface of human cells has a protease that is known as the type II transmembrane serine protease (TMPRSS2). As soon as the fusion occurs between the virus and the nasal lining cells, the TMPRSS2 removes the ACE2 while activating S proteins, which are spike-like proteins that are attached to the receptors. When these S proteins are activated, the structure of the membrane of the human cells is altered in such a way that allows for the entrance of the coronavirus. From what we have discussed so far, it is clear that the ACE2 receptors and TMPRSS2 protease are key in aiding the infection of human cells by the coronavirus.

Once inside the human cell, the coronavirus 2 will release its mRNA into the cytoplasm. This nucleic acid will then be translated into the nucleus of the host cell, producing all the parts, including the nucleocapsid, spike, and membrane proteins, that are required to assemble new viral entities. The nucleic acid of SARS-CoV-2 is easy to translate because it is mRNA which is a form of nucleic acid that is ready for translation into proteins. This is slightly different from viruses that have DNA as their nucleic acid. Such viruses would require transcription to mRNA before they can be translated into proteins. Having said this, the virus that causes COVID-19 takes over the infected cells at a faster rate as compared to DNA viruses. Many more copies of the viral nucleic acid are also made.

The viral structural and accessory proteins that are translated are then moved to the endoplasmic reticulum-Golgi intermediate compartment (ERGIC) of the host cell, where the viral assembling process commences. The nucleocapsid protein binds to the viral nucleic acid before moving to the ERGIC. The new viruses that are formed then move out of the infected cell through exocytosis in small vesicles. They will then infect more cells in the nasal lining through the same process. The exponential multiplication of the virus makes it easier for them to infect even more cells within a shorter period of time.

Possible Treatments

Treating infection by SARS-CoV-2 in the nasal cavity is assumed to help fight the virus before it establishes itself. Some of the methods that are being employed in an endeavor to destroy the coronavirus at the "nasal cavity" stage are (Cegolon et al., 2020; Sanders, 2020):

- nose spray to inactivate some of the viral proteins that are key to its infecting efficacy
- disinfectants used during surgeries for the sinuses
- diluted baby shampoo
- interferon alpha nasal spray, which interferes with the replication of the virus.

Some researchers are suggesting the use of nanobodies, which are specialized immune proteins obtained from alpacas, camels, and llamas. Nanobodies reportedly operate by covering the spike proteins on the virus, thereby inactivating them.

The Lungs and Immune System

The moment the coronavirus begins to attack the cells in the nasal cavity, the immune system of the body is triggered.

From the nasal cavity, the coronavirus will then spread to other parts of the respiratory system, especially the lungs. In the lungs, it can destroy even the tiny air sacs that are vital for air circulation. Most viruses cannot infect both the upper and lower respiratory tract. However, the coronavirus does, which is one of the reasons why it is quite dangerous. When SARS-CoV-2 destroys the air sacs, it significantly reduces the oxygen capacity of the lungs because 99% of the surface area of the lungs is attributed to the air sacs. Simply said, the survival of human beings is highly dependent on the effective functioning of these air sacs. They are the ones that provide the bloodstream with the oxygen that the body needs while excreting the carbon dioxide that is released by cells after metabolizing.

In the same way that the virus infects cells in the nasal cavity and uses them to replicate itself, it does so in the alveoli, that is, the air sacs. As the coronavirus continues to replicate and multiply in the lungs, they progressively destroy them. On the other hand, the alveoli are a harbor for macrophages, which are immune cells. Macrophages are always present in the air sacs to fight against any invaders that enter the lungs, smoke and microorganisms included. Therefore, when the coronavirus infects the lungs, the macrophages fight it. This implies that the first response to the coronavirus by the immune system is made by macrophages.

Sometimes, the macrophages might overpower the virus and destroy it, though this is not always the case. The virus may override the efforts of the macrophages to destroy it. In such cases, other immune cells, called the neutrophils, may intervene. When the activities of the virus overwhelm the efforts of the immune system, it may end up directing much of its resources toward fighting the virus. While the aim is to destroy the virus, the 'overreaction' by the immune system might cause more harm than good, especially to the lungs. This situation of an overzealous immune system is often referred to as the cytokine storm.

If the cytokine storm takes place in the lungs, then the lungs will suffer a double attack—from the coronavirus and the immune system. This alone destroys the air sacs. Moreover, during the cytokine storms, white blood cells release chemokines, which are inflammatory molecules. Chemokines invite more cells of the immune system to assist in fighting against the virus. As this happens, fluids and pus are produced, and these fill the air sacs, thereby blocking the transfer of both oxygen and carbon dioxide. Others suggest that fluids begin to flow from the blood vessels into the air sacs during the cytokine storm (Oh and Klivans, 2020). As a result, the body cells are deprived of the oxygen that they need while they fail to get rid of the carbon dioxide from respiratory processes. This situation in the lungs is what causes symptoms of breathlessness.

Hypoxia and Pneumonia

Hypoxia refers to a state where the amount of oxygen in the tissues is significantly reduced. Different tissues of the human body receive their oxygen from the blood, as it circulates to all parts of the body through a network of blood vessels. The blood gets this oxygen from the lungs. Normally, well-oxygenated blood should have an oxygen saturation range between 95% and 100%. When the amount of oxygen in the blood falls below 92%, then this becomes a cause for concern (Boston University, 2020) because the tissues will be on the verge of approaching a state of hypoxia. It has been established that as COVID-19 progresses and the coronaviruses continue to destroy the lung tissue, the risk of hypoxia increases.

Pneumonia is a condition where the air sacs of the lungs are inflamed. Pneumonia is also characterized by a scenario where the air sacs are clogged with fluid and pus. This greatly reduces the oxygen capacity of the lungs. Other symptoms that accompany pneumonia are cough, fever, shortness of breath, chills, fatigue, and pain in the chest. Pneumonia is one of the main conditions that are associated with coronavirus disease. This is why COVID-19 was originally called novel coronavirus-infected pneumonia (NCIP). From what I have explained about pneumonia, you can deduce that pneumonia can be a causative factor for hypoxia.

All tissues and organs of the human body require enough oxygen to keep their cells alive and functioning properly. This implies that limited availability of oxygen may cause some organs to malfunction—if they do not stop working completely. Some of the organs that have been reported to be affected in COVID-19 patients include the kidneys and heart. Severe cases of hypoxia may even cause irreversible damage.

There are various theories that are provided by researchers with regard to how the infection of the lungs with coronavirus causes hypoxia. First, it is believed that blood vessels constrict as they pass through parts of the lungs that are damaged due to, say, infection. This is meant to reduce blood flow toward those damaged areas and reduce the chance of transporting less oxygenated blood to the tissues. This is what should happen under normal circumstances, but it has been reported that in COVID-19 patients, the opposite is true. The blood vessels do not constrict but dilate even more. As a result, more blood will be oxygen-deficient as it passes through the damaged lung tissue whose surface area would have been reduced by the destruction of alveoli. Therefore, this blood will transport oxygen-deficient blood to the tissues, causing a state of hypoxia.

Another suggested theory is based on the formation of blood clots in the blood vessels of patients that have been infected by the coronavirus. It is suggested that the lining of the blood vessels may be inflamed along with the lung tissue that is damaged in COVID-19 patients. This may result in small blood clots forming in the blood vessels. Although it is assumed that such blood clotting may cause hypoxia, it is unlikely to be effective in doing this on its own. The levels of hypoxia that are reported in COVID-19 patients cannot be reached if blood clotting were the only factor to be considered. In other words, blood clotting may cause hypoxia if it is coupled with other factors that promote the condition.

The activities of the coronavirus in the lungs also disrupt the normal air-to-blood flow ratio that promotes proper oxygenation of body tissues. The efficient provision of enough oxygen to the tissues greatly relies upon the ventilation and perfusion of the alveoli. Ventilation is defined as the flow of oxygen in and out of the air sacs. Perfusion describes the flow of oxygen from the air sacs to the capillaries in the alveoli. In COVID-19 patients, ventilation and/or perfusion may be altered, thereby affecting the amount of oxygen that reaches the tissues.

Possible Treatments for Pneumonia

When a COVID-19 patient exhibits pneumonia symptoms, health professionals may recommend pain relievers to address the fever. If they are coughing, cough medicine may also be of help. However, in serious cases where the patients fail to breathe well, they have to be hospitalized so that they can utilize aided breathing facilities.

Possible Treatments for Hypoxia

Hypoxia is a serious condition that may have devastating effects on the human body. For example, extreme and elongated periods with the condition may aid brain damage. Other symptoms such as confusion, dizziness, seizures, and even stroke that are evident in COVID-19 patients are thought to primarily result from hypoxia. It is recommended that patients receive treatments that help to manage the situation of hypoxia to avoid even worse scenarios.

1. **Oxygen nasal cannula**: For patients with mild hypoxia, the oxygen nasal cannula is one of the most commonly used methods. This method is cost-effective, easy to use, and the technique is less complicated compared to other methods. It is also more preferred for the minimum aerosol generation that is associated with using it. It is also reported that it reduces the spread of COVID-19 in patients (Jiang and Wei, 2020). However, the disadvantage of this method is that it can only provide up to 40% of inspired oxygen. Moreover, since it requires that the oxygen be humidified in cases where oxygen flow is

above six liters per minute, the oxygen nasal cannula is less effective in severe hypoxia scenarios.

2. **Helmet ventilation**: Sometimes, non-breathing oxygen face masks are used to provide oxygen therapy in people with hypoxia. However, this method has its own disadvantages that are addressed by helmet ventilation. Unlike oxygen face masks, helmet ventilation is less prone to leakage of oxygen. The probability of aerosol spreading of the coronavirus is also lowered when helmet ventilation is used. However, challenges with helmet ventilation include difficulty in humidification and the requirement for high oxygen amounts since over 100 liters per minute of gases is required.

3. **High-Flow Nasal Oxygenation (HFNO)**: The HFNO therapy is effective for addressing severe cases of hypoxia before invasive methods are employed. This method is used to deliver warm and humidified oxygen into the body. The maximum possible flow rate that is feasible for this method is 70 liters per minute, which is quite huge compared to that for the oxygen nasal cannula. Other factors that make HFNO a good choice for managing hypoxia are

that it is more comfortable and relatively easy to tolerate.

4. **Mechanical ventilation**: This is a conventional method that even some patients who would have used other methods end up using. Mechanical ventilation involves the insertion of a mechanical ventilator for tracheal intubation. However, it has been reported that the mortality rate after intubation is quite high (Jiang and Wei, 2020). This makes methods such as HFNO more preferable. However, some suggest that the high mortality that results from mechanical ventilation might be because of late intubation.

5. **High Frequency Jet Ventilation (HFJV)**: This is a more advanced method that is coupled with an open system, reasonable tidal volumes, and lower pressures in the airway passages. The respiratory frequency that is provided by the HFJV is high and similar to that of the heart. With all these characteristics, HFJV is trusted to treat hypoxia in COVID-19 patients with increased efficiency.

An improved version of the HFJV is also available. This is called high frequency two-way jet ventilation (HFTJV). The additional feature of this method, as compared to the regular HFJV, is that it has inspiratory and expiratory phases. Injection of the jet pulse into the lungs marks the inspiratory phase, while the active discharge of the jet pulse is the expiratory phase. The expiratory phase helps to further reduce unnecessary pressures in the airway passages, in addition to improving the circulatory function in a way that imitates normal breathing processes.

Acute Respiratory Distress Syndrome

COVID-19 patients who suffer from coronavirus-related pneumonia are more likely to have acute respiratory distress syndrome (ARDS). ARDS is caused by the accumulation of fluid in the alveoli, leading to compromised transfer of oxygen to the bloodstream and the tissues. ARDS also causes carbon dioxide to build up in the tissues and bloodstream since the lungs become less capacitated and unable to play their role in excreting carbon dioxide. Severe cases of ARDS may ultimately lead to organ failure.

Some of the symptoms that are associated with ARDS are labored and frequent breathing as a result of shortness of breath, fever, tiredness, rapid pulse rate, mental confusion, and low blood pressure.

Possible Treatment for ARDS

There are different strategies that can be employed in treating ARDS:

1. **Oxygen capacitation**: Efforts to treat ARDS are mainly aimed at increasing the oxygen capacity of the lungs and possibly reducing the accumulation of fluid and pus in the air sacs. The purpose of all this is to save the patient from organ failure. Therefore, the interventions that are more appropriate for patients with ARDS are those that will aid their breathing and provide tissues with the oxygen that they require. Methods such as the ones that have been described for treating hypoxia can also be used in this case.

2. **Balancing fluids**: Another strategy to deal with ARDS is to manage fluids in the body. The idea is to reduce fluid collection in the lungs. When there are excess fluids in the body, the fluid levels in the air sacs may also increase. On the other hand, depriving the body of fluids might reduce fluid accumulation in the alveoli but may strain other organs such as the heart.

3. **Medication**: People with ARDS can be given medication that relieves the side effects of the condition. For example, they can be given pain relievers to reduce the discomfort that comes with ARDS. Blood thinners may also help to avoid the formation of blood clots in the lungs.

Recovery

The complications that are linked with coronavirus disease make it difficult for people to understand what recovery from this disease really entails. However, there are variations in the way people recover from COVID-19. Such variations are influenced by factors such as the extent to which one was affected by the coronavirus. Some effects are more severe and hence, more difficult to recover from. However, it is crucial to understand that it is completely OK not to feel as vibrant as you were before infection, even a few weeks after the isolation period. This is absolutely normal, especially with COVID-19.

Let's briefly look at what to expect when recovering from mild, moderate, and severe COVID-19 sickness:

- **What is recovery from mild COVID?**: Approximately 80% of people that are infected with the coronavirus may show mild to no symptoms at all. For those that exhibit mild symptoms, their recovery is relatively quick—usually between a week and 10 days. In fact, the recovery from mild COVID is similar to that of other respiratory infections such as influenza.

- **Recovery from moderate COVID?**: Symptoms of moderate COVID are more serious compared to those for the mild form of the disease. Most of the people that experienced mild symptoms of COVID-19 might have been admitted to the hospital for some time. Recovery takes longer for this group of individuals—up to several weeks. During their recovery, survivors of mild COVID may still experience moments of shortness of breath, fatigue, and/or coughing. The experiences vary with individuals.

- **Recovery from severe COVID**: People who ended up in the ICU or on ventilation aids are the ones that experienced severe COVID. This group of people sustained great injuries from the illness, including damage to some organs. Their recovery is normally the longest as it doesn't take anything less than several weeks to even months. The longer timeframes for the recovery of severe COVID-19 patients is due to the fact that the rejuvenation of damaged organs may take a long time. It, however, depends on the extent of the damage caused.

Possible Treatments

Some of the symptoms that may be experienced during the recovery phase of COVID-19 progression may be quite uncomfortable. Some medication to relieve pain may come in handy when you experience headaches and fevers. Some exercises and a proper diet enhance quick recovery, too. We will discuss more about the interventions that you might consider when COVID symptoms persist, even long after infection.

Chapter 3: Behaviour Change and Control Over Thoughts

Long COVID can have serious effects on your thoughts, and ultimately, your behavior. The trauma of the experience that you went through in the hands of the virus may take a long time to erase from your mind. It might continue to be vivid, as though it happened yesterday. You might feel like you cannot think straight—like your thoughts are being controlled from elsewhere. The anxiety and fear of another attack might stick around for longer than expected. Do you wonder when this 'madness' will disappear?

Well, it might not, but you might choose to outlive it. Just the fact that you survived the hospitalization is enough reason to encourage you that you can survive long COVID too. This chapter will provide you with some tips on effective positive behavior change and how to assume better control over your thoughts.

Create a Conducive Environment for Recovery

Your ability to properly recover highly depends on the environment that is available for your recovery. An unconducive environment can even worsen the psychological effects that are caused by COVID-19. In this section, we will discuss how you can create an environment that enhances quicker recovery from the long-term symptoms of coronavirus disease.

Limit COVID-Related Statistics

With the different waves of coronavirus infection emerging, in addition to the experience that you had during your hospitalization, the fear and anxiety associated with the pandemic might be difficult to deal with. This is especially true when you keep feeding your mind with dreadful information and statistics about COVID-19. What you constantly put into your mind is what creates your mindset, which eventually manifests as behavior. Hearing more about the exponential deaths that are caused by coronavirus disease does not create the right aura for your recovery.

It is crucial to note that you cannot completely shut your ears to the world and live as an island. You need information to make informed decisions, but you can sieve out information that is possibly toxic to your well-being. At this point, your mind is sensitive and vulnerable to damage by information that takes you down the memory lane of your experiences with COVID-19. Therefore, you need to be careful concerning the channels you watch on your television, the groups you join on social media, and even what you read. Feed yourself with information less related to the COVID-19 pandemic unless the information will encourage you to fight on and reclaim your identity.

Customize Your Physical Space

What speaks to your personality? Could it be flowers, music, silence, bright or dull colors? Whatever it is that makes you feel more at home plays a crucial role in aiding positivity in your thoughts and behavior. Create an environment that connects to your inner being. This also speeds up the recovery process.

You should also ensure that your physical space is well-ventilated for proper air circulation. Sanitizers, as well as soap and running water, should not be far-fetched, especially if you are sharing spaces with other people, say, family members.

Build a Support Network

Kristin Armstrong, an Olympian bicycler, once said, "The best thing to do when you find yourself in a hurting or vulnerable place is to surround yourself with the strongest, finest, most positive people you know." The people that Kristin was referring to are what I call a support network. You need people that encourage you to keep going when the going gets tough. These are the people that can be your source of strength when you feel weak and overwhelmed with negative thoughts. I call this "borrowed positivity," which is the resilience that you derive from your association with others. Borrowed positivity can help you to develop your personal resilience that can remain even when your support network is unavailable for any reason.

The Art of Creating a Support System

While creating a support network is of paramount importance, mistakes in the process may be costly. Mistakes such as incorporating the wrong people in your support system may not fulfill the intended purpose, which is to support you in building positivity. Build the right, positive support system. For that reason, this section is intended to give you recommendations on how to create your own support network and rebuild positivity within yourself.

1. **What is the problem?** First, you need to identify the problem that you want your support network to help you solve. There should be a gap that they can fit in if they are going to be effective. In this case, you might be experiencing bouts of low self-esteem, stress, anxiety, fear, and other emotions that are associated with negativity. Knowing the reason why you need a support group helps you to determine the people that should be in your support group.

2. **Who should be in your support system?** This question seems easy to answer, but this is the trickiest part of creating a support network during long COVID recovery. As I mentioned earlier, a wrong move here can jeopardize the whole intention of building a support system. There are basically three types of people that you should consider incorporating into your support network:

   - First, you should include those that you know and have long-standing relationships with, like family and friends. This group of people might not have any special expertise, but their love and care can push you more toward positivity. Your family and friends know you better and therefore know how to assist you best.

- Second, you should consider including people that have relevant professional expertise, even though they are not necessarily part of your social circles. These include doctors, nurses, psychologists, and life coaches. These people will offer you professional advice that is relevant to what you are going through. Your family and friends can even help you to reach out to these experts if need be.

- The third group is made up of people that you do not know but have experiences that are similar to yours. These could be people that have conquered the negativity that emanates from the journey through COVID illness or those that are currently going through experiences. Ideas that are shared by people who have walked down the same path as you are more effective. You feel like they understand what you are going to need from others. You should be willing to open up concerning your thoughts and feelings.

3. **Are you prepared to have them on board?** Now that you know who should be part of your support network, you might need to approach them. However, before you do that, you need to be ready for them. The people that you have chosen to be part of your support network are coming to help you, but are you ready to be assisted? Do you feel you can let them play their roles without your interference? You need to have a submissive attitude that acknowledges that you do not know everything, which is why feelings enable your support network members to help you.

4. **Can you approach them?** There are some members of your support system who are automatically present, even if you do not approach them for the task. Family and friends are such examples. If you are taken to the hospital for an illness, doctors will attend to your situation in a general manner. To them, it is like duty calls. However, when you privately approach them (by appointment) and open up to them, they can attend to your situation with a more customized approach. This way, they can help you better. For other support groups with people that you might not even know but have similar situations, make an effort to join them. If there is a need to

subscribe financially, you can also do so. You can find such support platforms even on social media. For example, there is a Facebook page called "Long Covid Support" where long COVID patients and other groups such as researchers can collaborate. You can learn much from such groups.

Implement the Law of Attraction

The Law of Attraction is a philosophy that is based on the belief that "like attracts like." This philosophy implies that positive thoughts attract positive things in life, including success, health, and opportunities for betterment. According to the Law of Attraction, thoughts release energy to the universe. Therefore, each thought vibrates at a certain frequency. When they are released into the universe in the form of energy, each thought will attract things that vibrate at the same frequency as itself to you. In that manner, positive thoughts will attract positive and more satisfying results, while negative thoughts yield negative and less desirable results.

This explanation that I have just given about the Law of Attraction implies that the same law applies both positively and negatively. How to apply it is then a matter of choice on your side. If you desire to achieve positive results, you should align your thoughts toward the positivity that will bring you the results that you want. Long COVID might have affected your perceptions, thoughts, and even behavior, but you can change that if you set your mind toward positivity. When negative thoughts emerge to say, for example, "I have wasted a lot of time being bedridden, and my business will die," tell yourself, "Thank God I have been able to survive this infection. I will work hard and revamp my business."

Principles of the Law of Attraction

There are three principles that govern the Law of Attraction. We have already explored one of them, which states that **like attracts like**. Let's explore the other two of these principles.

The second principle assumes that **nature abhors a vacuum**. According to this principle, the negative things, thoughts, and emotions in your life take up space for positive things. Therefore, you should drive out the negative things to create space for positive ones. Once you drive away negative things from your life, there is vacant space that you can fill in with positive ones if you decide to. Do not let thoughts about COVID-19 run your life. Drive them out and replace them with more positive thoughts that give you more energy toward improving your life.

The third principle says that **the present is always perfect**. This principle implies that there is always a better version of the present moment. It suggests that your idea of the present flawed moment is a matter of choice. Instead of focusing on what is wrong with the present moment, you can choose to concentrate on what you can do to make the present moment better. Instead of spending time wailing about your unpleasant experiences with COVID-19, focus on your recovery and the goals that you intend to achieve once you fully get back on your feet. You can certainly do it! All you need is affirmation from yourself.

How It Works

How you think affects your behavior. This is because what you think influences your feelings and emotions, both of which ultimately determine your behavior. Therefore, when you are able to control your thoughts toward positivity, you can also influence better and more productive behavior. For instance, if you complain less and focus more on recovering, you are more likely to do things that enhance your health.

Here are some steps that you can follow to implement the Law of Attraction as you recover from long COVID:

1. Decide What You Want

It will be very difficult to apply the Law of Attraction when you are not certain about your desires. Obviously, one of the things that you desire is regaining your health. You might have other goals that you would want to achieve after you recover. For instance, you might want to start a new business or upgrade the one you currently have. Or maybe you simply want to live long enough to see your grandchildren. You have to be clear on your desires if you want the Law of Attraction to work for you.

2. Learn the Art of Gratitude

It is unfortunate that most of us allow our minds to dwell on the "pains and unfairness" of life. Do you know that life appears the way you see it? It depends on the lens that you are using to view it. The same situations that can be viewed as painful can also be viewed as an opportunity to build up resilience. The inner strength that you had before COVID-19 struck cannot be compared to what you have now. You are better than before. Physical strength and health are things that you can regain.

Learn to look at positivity in situations. That is the only way you can cultivate the culture of gratitude within you. You were terribly sick, that is true and sad, but you are still alive and recovering from long COVID. There are millions of people that were hospitalized and so many never had the opportunity to come back home. Be grateful for the people that are taking care of you, the texts to check up on you that you always receive, and the food on your table. Appreciate each breath. Remember how costly each breath was when you were on the ventilator. The more grateful you are, the better positioned you are to receive good things from the universe.

3. Guard Your Words

You can lock yourself in negativity, illness, and hopelessness by the words you say about yourself and to yourself. Your self-talk should focus more on positivity. Do not say the things that you do not want to receive because that is what you will get. For example, when you're focused on your sickness, you might say, "This illness is staying for too long. I am tired." Instead, you could focus your concentration on healing and say, "Where I am coming from is further than where I am going. My recovery will soon be complete." The first statement is a voice of a person who is wallowing in failure and hopelessness, while the second one sounds like the one of an individual that is ready for a positive turnaround of things. Develop a habit of speaking positively about situations, even in the worse ones. If you do this, not even long COVID can hold you back.

4. Work on What You Want

Thinking positively and making positive affirmations are good because they orient you toward positivity. However, to achieve your desires, you should stand up and work toward them. Seek advice, build support networks, eat well, and exercise appropriately. Wake up and make your dreams a reality!

Meditation

Another way to enhance positivity is by practicing meditation. By definition, meditation refers to a set of techniques that train your mind to develop a healthy sense of perspective and heightened awareness. Meditation is based upon the fact that thoughts are always running through your mind. Therefore, it helps you to be more aware of your thoughts and thinking patterns but withholding any judgments. As a result, you understand your thoughts better, making it easier for you to control them. Symptoms such as anxiety, fear, and low self-esteem can be alleviated through meditation.

Types of Meditation With Examples

There are different types of meditation that you can employ. However, for all types of meditation, the preparatory procedures are more or less the same. The first thing is to find a conducive space for your meditation session. This could be a room within your house, a place in your garden, a park, or any other place of your choice. Be sure to choose a space with minimal possible distractions and noise.

The time that you choose for your session also matters. For instance, if you have kids and choose to meditate in your house, early mornings before your kids wake up or late evenings when they are fast asleep could be ideal. You wouldn't want to hear one of them requesting a drink while you are deeply meditating. If you are going to meditate while sitting down, you might need to prepare a chair, mat, cushion, bench, or anything that will make your meditation session as comfortable as possible. Some also prefer to set a stopwatch to mark the end of their session. This helps to avoid frequently checking the time, which can be extremely distracting.

The various types of meditation fall into two major categories, namely, concentrative and mindfulness meditation.

Concentrative Meditation

Concentrative meditation refers to techniques that involve focusing on something while switching yourself off to everything else around you. This category of meditation is of help when, say, you need to shun negative thoughts and concentrate on positive ones.

Types of meditation that fall under concentrative meditation include the following:

1. *Mantra Meditation*

This involves repeating a certain word or sound as a way to enhance focus on meditation. The word that you repeat does not need to have a particular meaning. It could be just a sound like the common 'ohm.' A meaningful word also works. For example, you could repeat the word 'heal.' It might even end up feeling like you are calling healing to yourself, which is what you want anyway.

How to Practice

Choose a word, sound, or phrase that resonates with what you want, how you are feeling, and what you intend to achieve with the meditation session. Whatever you choose becomes your mantra. Repeat the mantra while sitting in a calm place of your choice. This will help you to experience an inner feeling of peace. When you recognize that your thoughts have wandered, simply acknowledge that and continue reciting your mantra. You can obtain the best results when you close your eyes. Once you are done with your session, simply open your eyes, stop the mantra, and reconnect to your environment before you leave your meditation spot.

2. Visualization Meditation

This is a form of meditation that involves creating a picture of what you want or intend to achieve in your mind. It is more like you create a visual of the things that you desire. For instance, if long COVID has thwarted your self-esteem, you can visualize yourself exhibiting high levels of self-confidence. The main principle behind visualization meditation is tricking the mind. Your mind cannot differentiate between real and imaginary situations. Therefore, when you soak yourself in imaginary success, it will assume that the success was real. As a result, 'happiness' hormones can be released.

How to Practice

While sitting down in a calm place, close your eyes and place your hands on your lap. Now, begin to see yourself achieving the dream that you thought long COVID had stopped. For instance, you could visualize your graduation from the university of your choice. See people applauding as you walk down the aisle with your graduation gown and hat on. Add some more life to the picture that you are seeing. Hear the soft music that denotes victory and the faint wind sweeping your gown as if to say, "Congratulations!" Imagine the eyes of your youngsters staring at you with sheer admiration, as well as the hope that they want to be like you one day. Imagine everything that you want to experience as if the event was happening live. When you are done, you can open your eyes.

Mindfulness Meditation

Mindfulness meditation involves being in the present moment, and it usually helps by giving the meditating individual a greater sense of openness, awareness, and acceptance. Stress, anxiety, and fear can be addressed using mindfulness meditation. Usually, mindfulness meditation is done by taking note of your thoughts but avoiding being judgmental. Visualization can also be incorporated in mindfulness meditation if need be. With mindfulness meditation, you are able to relieve yourself from self-blame and thinking that there is something that you could do to prevent yourself from being a victim of long COVID. Instead, you look at your situation with better acceptance of things that you cannot change while you gather the confidence to face the future and achieve your goals, your health being one of them. You cannot change the fact that you contracted COVID-19 and suffered health-wise, but now that you survived it, then what? You need to practice mindfulness meditation.

Let's delve into some examples of mindfulness meditation:

1. *Basic Mindfulness Meditation*

To practice basic mindfulness meditation, find a place that you would prefer for your meditation session. I would recommend that you close your eyes, though you may be more comfortable keeping them open. Begin by focusing on your breath. Breathe slowly for about 5 seconds. Hold your breath for 2 seconds before breathing out again slowly. The breathing procedure is only there to help you focus on your meditation procedure. Once you have temporarily disconnected yourself from the environment, you begin to focus on your thoughts. Whether you are thinking about why you have not been feeling well for so long or why your spouse succumbed to coronavirus disease, it is fine. Just acknowledge your thoughts, but don't judge them. Rather, accept and own them while focusing on the present moment.

2. *Loving-Kindness Meditation*

Loving-kindness meditation is usually done together with visualization meditation. This type of meditation involves giving yourself some love, followed by a ripple effect where you send love to other people apart from yourself.

How to Practice

Visualize yourself and then start showering yourself with positive energy and goodwill. Send yourself good wishes for things that you really want to experience in your life. For instance, you can say, "May you attain unending good health," or "May you recover speedily and live your dreams." You can say as many good wishes as you can. After some time, replace yourself in the visualization with other people. Begin to send positive energy and goodwill to those people. You will realize how good it feels to wish someone well. It is also part of your healing process.

Hypnotherapy

Hypnotherapy is a form of complementary medicine that helps people to attain a state of elevated awareness and suggestibility. When individuals are in such a state, they can easily take suggestions that are given to them. This way, suggestions can be used to transform negative behaviors while incorporating more positive ones.

There are many misinterpretations that many people have when it comes to hypnotherapy. One of the most common is that some think that hypnotherapy strips you of your ability to reason and act logically. This notion suggests that hypnotized people can be easily manipulated into doing things that they do not want. However, this is not true because an individual in the hypnotic state is, in actual fact, assembled to resist suggestions that they do not want. They remain aware of who they are and what they want.

Hypnosis is a game of the mind. It is based on the idea of giving desirable suggestions to the subconscious mind. Your mind is divided into two major sections—the conscious and the subconscious mind. The conscious mind is the one that is responsible for your reasoning abilities and other functions in the body that involve logic. The subconscious mind is where your behaviors are rooted. Therefore, hypnotherapy targets the subconscious mind in changing undesirable behaviors and thoughts. However, it is difficult, if not impossible, to access the subconscious mind with a fully awake conscious mind. This is where hypnotherapy comes in—to help lower the dominance of the conscious mind while increasing that of the subconscious mind. As a result, suggestions are directed toward the subconscious mind with less interference from the conscious mind.

For you to clearly understand the process of hypnosis, I will describe the three steps that are involved:

1. **Induction**: Every session of hypnotherapy begins with induction. This can be defined as the process during which you prepare your mind so that it gradually enters the hypnotic state. It is a stage that marks the transition from being highly connected to the environment to being more connected to your subconscious mind. Just before the induction period, the conscious mind is dominant over the subconscious mind. This gradually changes as the induction progresses, such that the conscious mind gradually becomes less dominant. There are many ways through which induction can be done. Some prefer to

use breathing exercises or focusing on a certain part of the ceiling, among other examples.

2. **Hypnotic state**: If induction is well done, you should be able to enter the hypnotic state. This is the state of high awareness and suggestibility. The reason why your mind is more susceptible to suggestions at this stage is that the subconscious mind would be dominant over the conscious mind. Therefore, the conscious mind has less interference with suggestions that are given to the subconscious mind. This is the time when positive affirmations that align with what you want are said. For example, the hypnotherapist could say, "Refuse to be afraid, but choose to be strong and face the future."

3. **Reconnection**: When you feel that you have finished your session, you can reconnect to the environment around you. However, when your hypnotic session is over, keep affirming the positive suggestions that you received during the hypnotic procedure.

Clinical Hypnotherapy

People dealing with various aspects of COVID-19 can use clinical hypnotherapy. In fact, many people now prefer this option to address problems that emanated from COVID-19, be it anxiety, fear, reduced self-esteem, among others. In clinical hypnotherapy, sessions are guided by professional hypnotherapists or psychologists. In this section, I will take you through a typical hypnotherapy session. Let's get started!

1. Create a conducive environment for the session. Find a comfortable place to lie on—a bed or couch will do. If there are special aromas that make you relax, you can use them, too. Soft music of your choice is also a great idea.

2. Now, lie down on your back. Fix your eyes on a point in the ceiling and keep them there. Listen to your favorite music playing in the background, and take in the great aroma in the room.

3. Allow every part of your body to relax. Start with your head, neck, shoulders, chest, and keep going down. Feel your body relax, and

your eyelids become heavy. Slowly close them and relax.

4. Begin to focus more on the environment inside than the one outside you. Allow yourself to explore your subconscious mind and redirect your life to what you desire.

5. Start giving suggestions to your subconscious mind. It's time to let go of all the fear, anxiety, uncertainty, and self-condemnation. It's time to release all the pain that you have endured in the hands of COVID-19. Take out the faintness and loss of hope. Let them go. Let them fly away. Create space for better things that you desire—your health, achieving your life goals, peace, and self-confidence. You are going to be healthy, even more than before. You will achieve your dreams and make it in life. You are confident and fearless. You are strong emotionally and physically.

6. Now, open your eyes and reconnect to the world around you. Carry the suggestions with you and consciously live them. Use the same suggestions for your morning and evening affirmations to reinforce them. Believe in the positivity of the whole process.

Protect Others

Sometimes, your healing is in protecting others. The satisfaction that comes with helping another person not to go through what you went through can go a long way in enhancing your recovery from long COVID. Moreover, such courteous acts have a soothing effect on your thought patterns. Instead of dwelling on the fear, anxiety, and depression that is associated with the coronavirus pandemic, your thoughts are geared toward fighting it together with others. This is a more positive mindset that can help you to release yourself from the "mindset imprisonment" that was caused by your coronavirus infection. Let's explore some of the ways through which you can protect others from contracting coronavirus while redirecting your thoughts toward positivity in the process.

Observe COVID-19 Regulations

Despite the fact that you are in the recovery stage, you still need to adhere to COVID-19 protocols. It is not well-established whether a person who has recovered from coronavirus disease can be successfully attacked again, but some studies suggest that there is a possibility for reinfection (Mozes, 2021). More interestingly, those who are reinfected are unlikely to show symptoms of the disease. Asymptomatic people can easily spread the virus unknowingly because they assume they are not infected. However, decide to make a difference by keeping your cloth mask on when you are in public, using the elbow greeting, washing your hands with soap and running water, regularly sanitizing, and disinfecting surfaces. Who knows, you might save a life?

Testify to Others

When COVID-19 was declared a global pandemic, millions of people didn't believe in the reality of the disease. Surprisingly, even after the disease has taken so many lives and caused a lot of harm, some people do not understand the severity of the risk that people are facing during the COVID era. When you feel comfortable doing so, you may talk about your experience with the disease to others so that they may hear from someone who has been a victim of the coronavirus. Just tell someone who will also tell someone.

Be Careful of Your Comments on Social Media

What you say is a reflection of the type of mindset that you have. Try to reflect positivity in your comments on social media. If you are used to posting negative comments, it might take some time to master this art. You might find yourself typing some negative words—if you do this, then delete them. That's the process, and you will get there. What is important is to purpose it in your mind to send positive vibes out there. Your positive comment might not help everyone, but it will certainly save someone.

Have you ever heard of the saying, "The good you do, you do it for yourself, and the bad you do, you do it for yourself?" Somehow, the positive vibes that you send to other people will manifest in your own life.

Check on Others

Due to the COVID-19 pandemic, people have become so comfortable with being checked on over the phone. Most people understand that being away from each other physically is one of the best gifts we can give each other in times like this. However, communication is still one of the powerful tools that keep us together. Just a voice call or message will give someone hope. Even though you are also recovering from long COVID, let someone recover together with you through your message of hope. Two are always better than one.

Chapter 4: Exercises—

Guidance and Benefits

After recovering from COVID, most survivors find it difficult to return to their normal activities, especially exercise. Long COVID symptoms such as feeling weak, dizziness, and mild confusion are some of the reasons that make reconnecting with exercising more complicated than before. At the same time, some conditions associated with long COVID, such as cardiopulmonary disease, can be better addressed by engaging in exercising activities. It is now well-known through reported research output that exercise betters cardiovascular, digestive, and mental health (Public Health England, 2016). On the other hand, inactivity, even to 'healthy' individuals, can cause negative health effects such as obesity.

It is even believed that the inactivity, especially due to national lockdowns due to the COVID pandemic, worsened the risk of COVID for some people. For example, individuals with chronic conditions such as obesity and hypertension likely got worse, even before they may have been infected by the coronavirus. It is also well-established that people with chronic conditions were at a higher risk of exhibiting more severe symptoms of COVID-19.

What Is Exercise?

There is a misconception that exercise is all about sports. People can exercise without necessarily engaging in sporting activities. Exercise refers to any physical activity that involves the release of energy. From this definition, walking, gardening, or cleaning the house are all forms of exercise. Sprinting, playing football, and lifting weights are also exercises. Some exercises are more intense than others.

When time frames for doing the exercises are considered, intense and less vigorous exercises may yield similar results. For example, 150 minutes of moderate exercise, coupled with some muscle-strengthening exercises, can be as good as 75 minutes of intense exercise that is equally accompanied by exercises for the muscles (Samlan et al., 2021). Moderate exercise increases the breathing rate, yet one can still talk without difficulty while doing it. In vigorous exercise, it is difficult to talk.

Some people prefer to have scheduled sessions of exercise. This is a great idea because it binds them to follow their schedules, thereby enabling them to exercise regularly. Some would rather exercise when they feel like it. While this is good because they work out when they are emotionally and mentally ready, it may also lead to a more relaxed approach toward exercise. Another easy way to exercise is to replace some technology with manual completion of tasks. For instance, you might choose to walk to the nearest shops, rather than using a car. Instead of using the elevator to go up to your office each morning, you might opt to use the stairs. You can even create fun out of exercising! One example of incorporating fun into your exercising procedures is dancing, although it is often overlooked.

Benefits of Exercise

While exercise is important to people who are suffering from long COVID, it is important to note that an abrupt return to intense exercise can cause more harm than good. Individuals need to learn methods that enhance a safe return to exercise routines. It is crucial to check the specific condition of the COVID survivors during their time of recovery. The reason for this is that there are some conditions that can worsen an individual's health situation if exercise is undertaken. Let's look at myocarditis, for example. Myocarditis is a condition of the heart where its ability to pump blood is compromised. Abnormal heart rhythms are another symptom of myocarditis. People suffering from myocarditis are not recommended to engage in exercising activities because doing that is associated with higher mortality rates. People who were hospitalized for COVID-19 might have suffered from viral myocarditis, and exercising can increase their probability of heart failure. Therefore, people that are recovering from this condition should not exercise.

The Risk Stratifying Approach

You might then be wondering how one knows if they are supposed to engage in exercising or not. It is recommended that you approach your doctor or other health experts for professional advice before starting your exercise routines. They will use what is called the risk stratifying approach to analyze your safety after doing exercises. Here are the questions that can help health professionals to give you advice as to whether you should commence with exercise routines or not.

Did You Show Symptoms of COVID-19?

Some people do not show serious symptoms of COVID-19 for at least 7 days, while some show various symptoms that differ in their combinations and severity. In this case, I am referring to symptoms that result in hospitalization. Such symptoms can be categorized as follows:

- **Cardiac symptoms**: This category includes symptoms like breathlessness, chest pain, palpitations, as well as temporary unconsciousness that results from an abnormal fall in blood pressure.

- **Adverse psychological symptoms**: Severe anxiety, intense stress, and even physical symptoms such as nausea are examples of adverse psychological symptoms, especially if they lead to post-traumatic stress disorder (PTSD). The condition of PTSD is usually experienced by most people who survive a certain type of danger, and COVID-19 is certainly not an exception.

- **Enduring symptoms**: These could be symptoms that affect the respiratory, cardiovascular, and gastrointestinal systems. Rheumatological symptoms attack the joints, ligaments, and muscles.

If you did not exhibit symptoms like the ones that I have mentioned, then it is unlikely that COVID-

19 affected your ability to exercise. In that case, you can employ a phased return to exercise. I will explain more about the phased return later in this chapter. If you showed symptoms that had to be treated in the hospital, then caution has to be taken to preserve your health and life. There might be a need to assess the type of symptoms that you experienced.

Were You Hospitalized for COVID-19?

There are two classes of people that showed symptoms for coronavirus disease—those that were hospitalized for symptoms and those that were not. If you were hospitalized for certain COVID symptoms, such as the ones that we discussed earlier, your ability to return to exercise should be assessed and recommended by health professionals. The first step that you should take is to avail yourself of COVID-19 rehabilitation services from your local hospital. This will help you to get appropriate assistance while you recover. If the symptoms that you exhibited did not lead to admission to the hospital, your return to phased exercise activities is safer, but caution needs to be taken by considering the type of symptoms that you experienced.

What Are the Symptoms That You Experienced?

This question is very important for individuals that were never hospitalized for coronavirus disease yet showed some symptoms. By the way, not all COVID sufferers were hospitalized because they appeared fit enough to avoid a hospital stay. That is why there are still people that died of COVID in their homes. One of the reasons why it is crucial to relook at the symptoms that individuals showed is to ensure that they receive the right recommendations concerning exercises. Mind you, different symptoms of COVID-19 have unique correlations with exercise.

- **Cardiac symptoms without hospital treatment**: In the event that you were not admitted to the hospital but showed cardiac symptoms, more assessments should be done before you can start exercising again. This might require professional advice from cardiology experts. To ensure that you get the appropriate advice, you might need to go through cardiopulmonary exercise testing, specialist blood panel, electrocardiography, or echocardiography.

The cardiopulmonary exercise test, which is also called the oxygen consumption test, assesses your ability to do exercises. This is done by collecting information about your lungs and heart to see if their response to exercise is either normal or abnormal. The specialist blood panel involves a series of tests that analyze your blood composition, including cholesterol, glucose, carbon dioxide, urea nitrogen levels, and also electrolytes. Electrocardiography is a technology that measures the electrical energy of your heart while you are not exercising. Your heart rate and rhythm, as well as conditions such as hypertension and previous cases of heart failure, can be detected using electrocardiography. Echocardiography is another advance in technology that assists doctors to better assess the state of your heart and its valves. This technology involves using sound waves to produce a live image of the heart of a patient. Therefore, doctors can even detect blood clots in the chambers of the heart through echocardiography.

If cardiac assessments that are carried out show you have myocarditis, then you should refrain from exercising for a period between 3 and 6 months while you periodically go for a checkup to monitor your healing progress. If you have no myocarditis but show that you have other heart-related conditions, you should take part in a rehabilitation session at your local hospital. It is not advised for you to exercise with such conditions.

Not all people that were hospitalized for COVID were showing the same symptoms. The disease affected people's health in different ways, depending on other factors. For example, individuals that had underlying health conditions were usually affected to a greater extent.

- **Adverse psychological symptoms, but no hospitalization**: Some people do not exhibit any cardiovascular symptoms but may show intense psychological symptoms. Are you one of such people? If yes, then you should seek assistance from your local psychological services. The services that you might need are cognitive behavioral therapy or desensitization and reprocessing of eye movement. Cognitive behavioral therapy sessions help you drive away negative thoughts and perceptions that might have emanated from infection by the coronavirus. This therapy also assists you in dealing with emotions such as fear, anxiety, and depression. After sessions of cognitive behavioral therapy, you can recover positivity toward yourself, others, and the world around you. Similarly, the eye movement desensitization and reprocessing (EMDR) procedure will help you to address the negative emotions and thoughts that are associated with your experience with COVID-19. Part of this procedure requires you to recall the event that caused distress before the therapy that involves eye movements is conducted. After your rehabilitation process through cognitive behavioral therapy and/or EMDR, you can return to physical activity in a phased manner.

- **Other enduring symptoms**: This category includes people that did not show either cardiac or psychological complications from infection by the coronavirus. However, these people experienced long-standing effects in their bodies, particularly on the respiratory, gastrointestinal, and skeletal systems. If this category describes you best, engage with your local COVID-19 rehabilitation service providers near you. It is risky to exercise without seeking professional recommendations as exercise may worsen your condition.

Phased Return to Exercises

The phased return to exercise is an approach that is meant to help your body gradually adapt to physical activity after the damage that was caused by COVID-19. It is the recommended way to safely return to exercise routines with less possibility of further harming your body. In this section, I will explain the phases that you should go through as you gradually resume physical activity.

As I explain, I will also refer to the rate of perceived exertion (RPE). This is a method of measuring the intensity of the physical activity that you engage in at any given time. This is done using the Borg scale, which has numbers ranging from 6 to 20. When there is no exertion at all, then the scale shows 6, whereas 20 represents a maximum effort in exertion. In other words, when you are lying down, the scale will show 6, whereas 20 can be equated to pushing a car against a steep hill. As the numbers on the scale increase from 6 to 20, your heart rate also rises. Other reports also showed that headaches are more common symptoms of coronavirus disease in people who are below the age of 65.

For each session of physical activity, you should take some time to warm up before you start and cool down after your session. This allows for a smooth transition between rest and exercising moments, thereby preventing your body from experiencing shock from rapidly switching between two extremities. You will repeat each phase consecutively for 7 days unless you feel that you are not ready to go to the next phase. It is not recommended for you to exercise when you haven't fully recovered from the previous day's exercises. The same applies when you notice returning or new symptoms showing up. Do not hesitate to seek medical advice when you notice abnormal breathing patterns. When you try a higher phase and realize that you cannot cope, you should go back a step lower until you feel that you are ready for the next phase.

Phase 1

In the initial phase, the RPE should not exceed 8. The main goal of this phase is to prepare your body to return to exercise. This is why the activity at this stage is mild to avoid shocking your body. At this stage, you should consider resting, stretching, gentle walking, as well as breathing and balancing exercises.

Phase 2

The intensity of physical activity at this phase is more than that of phase 1. However, it is still a low intensity level. Remember, you are gradually reintroducing your body to physical activity. The most appropriate activities at this stage are light household chores, light yoga, and walking. You can increase the time frame for your activities by 10 to 15 minutes each day or the 7 days of this phase. The RPE that is recommended for this stage is between 6 and 11, inclusive. When you feel that you can walk for 30 minutes without stopping, at an RPE of 11, then you can proceed to phase 3.

Phase 3

This phase is characterized by moderate strength and aerobic exercises. On day 1 in this phase, you can start with two sessions of aerobic exercises that run for 5 minutes each. The sessions should be separated by an interim block of recovery. For all consecutive days, you can add one more 5-minute interval if you feel you can tolerate it. This phase can be completed at an RPE between 12 and 14. You can only progress to the next phase of exercise when you have successfully adapted to exercising for 30 minutes and recovering well within an hour.

Phase 4

Just like in phase 3, phase 4 includes strength and aerobic exercises of moderate intensity. The only difference is that phase 4 additionally incorporates functioning and coordination skills as part of the exercises. It is recommended that you do these exercises for 2 days, followed by 1 day of recovery. You can continue to do this for 7 days if the fatigue levels are not abnormal. The suggested RPE range for this phase is 12 to 14.

Phase 5

The goal for this phase is to help you determine whether you can carry on with your normal physical activity as before infection by SARS-CoV-2. Simply said, this phase marks the baseline for your normal everyday exercises. This is why an RPE range that is above 15 is recommended for this stage. However, you can still increase the RPE gradually to make the transition more smooth.

Practical Exercises

With the knowledge that you have gained concerning your phased return to exercising, this section will provide you with practical exercise suggestions for each phase. The exercises that are given in this section are not exhaustive—there are many others that you can engage in. Therefore, if you are not comfortable with the ones provided in this section, you can always find others that you prefer more. However, I am confident that you will enjoy these exercises and find them helpful.

Phase 1 Exercises

Here are some of the exercises that you can do in phase 1:

The Quad Stretch

Follow the steps below to do the quad stretch.

- Find a conducive space for you to carry out your exercises.
- Stand on one leg, close to a wall or chair (if you feel that you cannot balance on your own).
- Lift your left foot toward your back so that your heel faces upward. Use your left hand to grab the top part of the foot that you have

lifted until your heel hits the back of your thigh. By this time, your knee should be pointing down toward the floor. While in this position, you should feel the front part of your leg stretching.

- Slightly move your thigh forward if you can tolerate the deeper stretch that results.
- Hold yourself in this position for an average of 20 seconds before switching your legs.
- You can repeat this procedure two to three times.

The Shoulder and Chest Stretch

As the name of the exercise suggests, this physical activity will help you to stretch your shoulder and chest area. Here is the procedure for the exercise:

- Stand and put your hands toward your back. Clasp them together without letting them touch the rest of your body. Be sure that both hands are straight.
- Now, gradually lift your hands toward the ceiling up to a position that you are comfortable with. Pay attention to your shoulders and chest—you should feel them stretch.
- Hold this position for approximately 20 seconds.

- Repeat the whole procedure three times.

Deep Breathing Activity

You are going to practice deep breathing. To make the activity mild, you will do the breathing exercise while lying on your back. Follow these steps:

- Prepare your space for the exercise. A bed, couch, mattress, or a floor with a mat can be more conducive for this activity. For the purpose of describing this procedure, I will assume you choose a mattress.
- Lie on your mattress, with your back toward it.
- Now, bend both knees until the soles of your feet are parallel to the mattress, with your knees pointing toward the ceiling.
- With your hands on top of your stomach, close your eyes to enhance your focus on the breathing exercise.
- While closing your lips, lift your tongue until it touches the top of your mouth.
- Inhale through your nose and allow the air to go into your stomach to the area that you are holding with your hands.
- Gradually breathe out through your nose.
- Repeat these deep breaths for not more than a minute.

Phase 2 Exercises

Remember, this phase still requires you to do mild exercises. Keep this in mind and avoid overworking your body against the phase of physical activity you are in. I have compiled some activities that you may consider in this phase, and these are:

Yoga

Enjoy some light yoga that is suitable for a person who engaged in little to no activity for a long time, especially due to sickness. This exercise will work out your hip and lower abdomen area. To do this exercise, follow these easy steps:

1. Lay your mat on the floor and lie down on it with your back facing toward the floor.
2. Bend your knees until your feet are completely flat on the mat.
3. Bring your hands to your sides and place them down onto the mat. Make sure your palms are parallel to the mat.
4. Slightly lift your pelvic area toward the ceiling as you inhale and then flatten it back onto the floor as you exhale. Repeat this step four or five times.
5. Begin to lift your pelvic area toward the ceiling again, but this time continue doing so until

your body is straight from your shoulders all the way to your knees. Your head, feet, and palms should remain on the mat. Hold this position for about 3 seconds.

6. Start to roll back down to the flat position in a gradual manner.

7. Repeat steps (6) and (7) three times, ensuring that your legs stick together.

8. Now, slowly drop your left leg toward your left side as much as is comfortable for you. Your right leg and the rest of the body should maintain their original position as you do so.

9. Bring the left leg back to its position while repeating step (8) but this time moving your right leg toward your right side.

10. Repeat steps (8) and (9) four times.

Deep Breathing Exercise

Follow this procedure:

1. Lie on your stomach and prepare a resting place for your head using your hands. This will help you to keep your nose from the mattress and allow you to breathe.

2. Close your eyes and lips. You can decide whether you are comfortable with placing your tongue on the roof of your mouth or not.

3. Take a deep breath through your nose and focus on how your stomach moves into the mattress.
4. Slowly breathe out. This can take up to 5 seconds, depending on your ability to slow down the exhale process.
5. Repeat the whole procedure for approximately 1 minute.

Phase 3 Exercises

In this phase, you are beginning to drift from more stationary exercises toward more active ones. I will direct you on how to do some mild aerobic and strength exercises.

Mild Jumping Jacks

Unlike the other exercises that we did in phases 1 and 2, jumping jacks will increase your heart rate. Your muscles will be at work, too. Let's get started!

1. Stand with your feet together and your hands on your sides.
2. Step to the right with your right foot. As you do this, bring your right arm up above your head. Your weight will slightly move to your left leg as you do this.

3. Return your right foot and arm back to the original position.

4. Quickly step out with your left foot toward the left side while lifting your left arm toward the top of your head. This step should immediately follow step (3) so that it looks like a continuation. Go back to your starting position.

5. Continue exchanging movements between your right and left foot as described in steps (3) and (4) as much as you can.

Squat and Hit

Do you want to have the feel of being a boxer? You can punch the air as you provide your heart and muscles with more action. Here is how to do it:

1. Stand with your feet apart—a bit wider than the shoulder-to-shoulder distance.

2. Your arms should be by your sides.

3. Squat in such a way that your knees protrude forward, your chest is up, and your butt is undoubtedly backward.

4. Stand up, and without completely straightening your legs, throw a cross-body punch into the air with your fists, one after the other.

5. Repeat steps (3) and (4) as many times as is possible for you.

Phase 4 Exercises

Here are some of the exercises that you can do in phase 4 of returning to exercises:

Wall Push-Ups

Wall push-ups are strength exercises. Such exercises, also called resistance exercises, are meant to increase your level of endurance. Enjoy your endurance training through push-ups by completing the following steps:

1. Find a wall or something strong that you can hold onto without it tipping over.
2. Stand against the wall and place your palms against it, with a shoulder distance between them. Make sure the distance of your feet from the wall allows you to slightly tilt over when your hands are stretched toward the wall.
3. As your arms bend, bring your chest toward the wall while you breathe in. Hold yourself in that position for 2 seconds.
4. Push yourself out as you breathe out.
5. Repeat the push-ups at least 10 times.

Jump the Rope

This exercise incorporates hand and foot coordination as part of the activity. All you need is a skipping rope. You can wear gym shoes if you have them, but any other sports shoes will work perfectly well.

1. Be sure to adjust the size of the rope to suit your height and to avoid falling over. To do this, stand on the middle of the rope with both feet. Now, extend the rope to your armpits. Mark that size because that is the one that is perfect for your height.
2. Begin to jog forward while swinging the rope over your head and under your feet. You should not step over the rope. Do this for 20 seconds.
3. Start jogging backward while moving your rope as described in step (2).
4. Rest for 125 seconds before starting another "forward and backward" set.
5. Repeat the whole procedure as many times as you can.

Phase 5 Exercises

Phase 5 exercises are similar to exercises for any healthy individual, so they can be used even after the recovery period is complete. In this phase, you can do aerobic exercises and strength exercises. Remember, aerobic exercises involve oxygen circulation. During such exercises, the heart and lungs are highly at work, and this improves the way they function. Strength exercises help to strengthen certain muscles of your body.

Coordination skills are also incorporated as they enhance mental health and mood. The contribution of coordination exercises to your mood is promoted by the production of "happy hormones," which are known as endorphins. Good coordination also reduces the probability of injuries during physical activity by enhancing flexibility and agility.

Many exercises fall into the phase 5 category, and these include the following:

- brisk walking
- cycling
- swimming
- rope skipping
- dancing

However, I will also suggest other exercises that you can try. Have fun with these while you are redirecting your body to physical activity.

Star Jump

The star jump is an exercise that joins aerobics and coordination acumen. There are a number of variations to this exercise that are meant to incorporate more fun into the activity. Here are the simple steps to the basic star jump exercise:

1. Stand with your feet together while your arms hang by your sides.
2. Jump and land with your feet spread out. The distance between your feet should be more than shoulder-to-shoulder length.
3. While you jump, your arms should move up toward the upper center of your head. The moment your feet hit the ground, clap your hands above your head.
4. Jump again to bring your feet and arms back to the original position.
5. Repeat the whole procedure as many times as you can without stopping.

Foot Tap

Try to do the slow version of this exercise and then start doing it faster.

1. Stand in a well-ventilated space.
2. Lift your right leg and bend it toward your left. It should be as if you want to touch the center

of your left thigh with the heel of your right foot.

3. Tap the inner side of your right foot with your left-hand fingers and place the leg down.
4. Now, lift the left leg and tap it with your right-hand fingers.
5. Repeat this slowly until you are well acquainted with the coordination aspect of the physical activity.
6. Begin to do the exercise faster while jumping when you lift a foot and landing as you tap the lifted foot with your fingers.

Chapter 5: Nutrition Guidance for General Illness Recovery

For adequate recovery from any form of sickness, you should build up a formidable immune system. Long COVID can put up a great fight against your immune system, but there is a lot that you can do to help it fight back. One of the most effective ways to equip your immune system is by watching what you eat. A healthy diet can boost your immune system, thereby enhancing your recovery, while a poor diet can further weaken it.

In this chapter, we will explore various aspects of nutrition and a stronger immune system. The overall idea is to hasten and strengthen your immune system. We will also look at a balanced diet and other foods that do not have a direct impact on your immune system, yet they do improve your recovery process.

Components of the Immune System

Before we start discussing what you should eat to enhance your immune system and enhance a quicker and smoother recovery, let us briefly explore what we are referring to as the immune system. Understanding the various components of the immune system will help you get the bigger picture when we start discussing the various foods and the nutrients that they contain in relation to boosting your immune system. There are two major components of the immune system that we are going to look at in brief.

1. Organs and Tissues

Your immune system is made up of different body parts that work together to ensure that your body is protected from infections. Two of the most important parts are the bone marrow and thymus. The thymus is responsible for the production of important cells in the immune system—lymphocytes. Two types of lymphocytes that exist are the B-lymphocytes and T-lymphocytes. So, the T-lymphocytes are the ones that move to the thymus, while the B-lymphocytes stay in the bone marrow for them to mature. In the thymus, the production of T-cells is completed with the help of the enzyme thrombin. The T-cells are further differentiated into helper T-cells and cytotoxic T-cells. Various proteins are expressed on the surface of T-lymphocytes, including CD8 and CD4 proteins.

When the B-cells and T-cells mature in the bone marrow and thymus, respectively, they move to the spleen and lymph nodes, where they can stay until their activity is required. In the spleen, blood is filtered such that healthy red blood cells pass while damaged ones are held and broken down by macrophages, which are white blood cells. Apart from storing white blood cells and platelets, the spleen helps the body to identify possibly infectious external objects and microorganisms.

Other important parts of the immune system are the gut-associated lymphoid tissues (GALT) and the mucosa-associated lymphoid tissues (MALT). MALTs are found in parts of the body that have mucosae, such as the mouth, eyes, skin, nose, and intestines. GALTs are found along the gastrointestinal tract, appendix, and tonsils. There are macrophages and lymphocytes present in these tissues to protect the body from being invaded by microorganisms.

2. Immune Cells

Apart from the body part, there are many other cells that put together their combined effort to protect the body. Cells enhance either innate immunity, which is non-specific, or adaptive immunity, which is specific. Immune cells are part of your blood, and they are usually known as leukocytes or white blood cells. The white blood cells in your blood can be divided into two categories, that is, granulocytes and lymphoblasts.

Granulocytes have granules in their cytoplasm, and these granules contain enzymes. Basophils, neutrophils, and eosinophils are all granulocytes. Neutrophils are part of the innate immune system, as they quickly respond to invaders in the body. Together with macrophages, they alert other parts of the immune system if there are any issues that arise from their response.

Lymphoblasts include cells that are involved in the adaptive immune system, such as the B-lymphocytes and natural killer T-lymphocytes. B-lymphocytes produce antibodies, while T-lymphocytes use cell-mediated responses in fighting pathogens.

A Balanced Diet

COVID-19 on its own is a disease that makes it difficult for you to eat even your favorite meals. Remember some of the symptoms of the disease—nausea, sore throat that makes it difficult to swallow food, loss of appetite, and even reduced to no senses of taste and smell. Some of these symptoms may persist as part of long COVID symptoms. Even though such symptoms and others may be a hindrance to eating properly, you should make it a point to eat a diet that will cater to your bodily needs while enhancing your recovery at the same time.

In this section, we will discuss more about a balanced diet. This refers to a diet that contains all the important nutrients in the right quantities. By right quantities, I mean that for each nutrient, there are certain amounts that are recommended, and those are the healthy amounts. As we discuss the balanced diet, you will also note that there are some nutrients that I will emphasize more than others. This is simply because the focus is on a balanced diet, but with more emphasis on foods that promote your recovery. Let's have a look at the components of a balanced diet first.

Components of a Balanced Diet

By "components of a balanced diet," I am referring to the various nutrients that your overall diet should include for it to be designated as balanced. It is important to note each nutrient has its own functions in the body, so in its absence, those functions are left unattended. So, let's explore what your meals should contain.

Macronutrients

Macronutrients are those that are required by the body in large quantities. This section will enlighten you on the different macronutrients that your body needs for you to recover well. We will also be highlighting some of the macronutrients that you should be on the lookout for because they can potentially cause more harm than good in your body.

1. Carbohydrates

Carbohydrates are important in hastening your recovery after a COVID-19 sickness, especially if you were hospitalized for the disease. They provide most of the energy that you need from your food. This means that carbohydrate-deficient foods may deprive you of the energy you need as you recover. You might, therefore, feel weak as a result. Whole wheat grains, cereals, potatoes, and rice are great sources of carbohydrates.

During the time when you lose your appetite and experience other symptoms of COVID-19, your body depends on the energy stored in the form of fat and glycogen in the muscles. Your body would be in a form of hibernation, but it can't stay like that forever. You need to re-boost your energy stores while providing your body with some to use immediately as you recover.

There are three types of carbohydrates that you should consider adding to your diet. These are:

- **Sugars**: This is the simplest form of carbohydrates. When consumed, sugar is quickly used up by the body, so it does not keep you feeling full for long. Glucose and fructose are both simple sugars.
- **Starches**: These are the main component in most staple foods. They are a complex form of carbohydrates made up of combinations of simple sugars.
- **Fibers**: These are also complex carbohydrates. Fibers can either be soluble or insoluble. Insoluble fibers help to enhance the smoother movement of food along the gastrointestinal tract. You can also stay fuller for longer periods.

Carbohydrates have the ability to reduce the number of cells that go through apoptosis (or self-destruction). Mind you, severe cases of COVID-19 may cause apoptosis of lymphocytes, which are an important part of the immune system. Therefore, eating a diet that has carbohydrates is good for your immune system.

In times of stress, which is comparable to what people experience during long COVID, people tend to alter their eating behaviors. For example, most people are inclined to eat more sugars than other types of carbohydrates. This can worsen their health condition because simple carbohydrates, like sugars, may cause metabolic syndrome, hyperglycemia, and type 2 diabetes when consumed in excess. Overconsumption of carbohydrates may also cause dysregulation of immune responses, which is what you do not want at this point.

Some experimental studies recommend not excluding carbohydrates from the diet but including them in reasonably low amounts for people with other underlying conditions such as diabetes. In one study, experiments that were done on mice demonstrated that a diet low in carbohydrates but high in fats could enhance protection against lethal influenza (Goldberg et al., 2019). On that note, this diet can help to reduce the severity of COVID-19 in diabetic patients. It is also suggested that it could help them to recover from long COVID as well.

2. Proteins

Proteins are mainly known as body-building foods. However, some of the amino acids from the proteins that you consume are part of important enzymes and hormones in the body. Due to their body-building abilities, proteins can also play a role in the repair of damaged cells and tissues in the body.

We discussed the cytokine storm in previous chapters. Just to help you recall, it is a hyper-inflammatory response that is accompanied by an over-release of cytokines as the immune system would be trying to fight the invasion by the coronavirus. This hyper-release of cytokines causes damage to many organs and might even trigger death. Although antiviral and anti-inflammatory medications help a lot in this case, amino acids from the proteins that you eat also contribute to reducing the rate at which the cytokines are released. This action, partly by amino acids, reduces the number of death cases that are attributed to COVID-19.

One of the amino acids that have been experimented on and reported to have positive effects on protecting the multi-organ dysfunction that is caused by coronavirus infection is L-glutamine (Nutrition and Diet, 2020). Reduced intake of glutamine through your diet reduces the differentiation of B-lymphocytes. This, in turn, reduces the production of antibodies against specific infections due to compromised differentiation of B-cells. Inadequate amounts of glutamine in the body also suppress the proliferation of T-cells, as well as affecting the function of other immune cells, including the macrophages.

If you were or are still experiencing nausea and vomiting, you might be deficient in proteins and calories by now. Symptoms of nausea, vomiting, and loss of appetite go hand in hand with the cytokine storm. If not attended to, such a situation can have detrimental effects on your overall health. However, the European Society for Clinical Nutrition and Metabolism (ESPEN) recommended that COVID patients and survivors should be given nutritional supplements as long as they can eat. ESPEN recommends that the patients should be given at least 30 grams of proteins every day to ensure that they recover well.

Other than modulating the immune system, proteins are also crucial for protecting your muscle mass due to infection by the coronavirus. It is reported that COVID-19 also negatively affects the metabolism of proteins. For example, muscle and protein breakdown increases, accompanied by reduced muscle synthesis and increased production of proteins that are required during the acute phase of COVID-19 (Nutrition and Diet, 2020).

A diet that is void of proteins and amino acids increases the body's susceptibility to infectious diseases. The body's first line of defense against pathogenic microorganisms is the physical barrier. The limited intake of protein has a negative impact on the physical barrier by reducing the thickness of the collagen and connective tissue. Moreover, the antibodies in the physical barrier are also reduced, and this makes it easy for an infecting agent to attack.

Some of the good sources of proteins are lean meats such as beef, kangaroo, and lamb. Bush birds, turkeys, and chicken are also rich in proteins. You can as well turn to seafood and fish for your protein sources. In that case, you can eat prawns, lobsters, clams, oysters, and crabs. You can also eat eggs or dairy products such as Greek yogurt, cottage cheese, and milk.

3. Fats

Most dietary fats are triglycerides. There are three major forms of fatty acids that you can obtain from a diet. These are monounsaturated, polyunsaturated, and saturated fats. Olive oil is a good source of monounsaturated fatty acids, while saturated fats are usually of animal origin. Nuts and seeds are great sources of polyunsaturated fatty acids. Monounsaturated and polyunsaturated fats are both regarded as healthy fats because they do not lead to the accumulation of bad cholesterol. On the other hand, saturated fats are less healthy. However, during recovery from sickness such as COVID-19, patients require all forms of fats to rejuvenate their calorie and energy stores. It is, however, important to note that too high an intake of fats is not recommended. It has been proven through experimental work that too high an intake of dietary fats causes intestinal changes that lead to increased permeability of the walls of the intestines. Overall, this change is reported to cause system inflammation that may affect the proper function of the immune system (Wypych et al., 2017).

Some of the vitamins that are important in boosting your immune system are lipid-soluble, so fat deficiency may hinder the transportation and function of such vitamins. For instance, vitamins A, D, E, and K are fat-soluble vitamins, and your immune system needs them. Dietary fats also contribute to the maintenance of the integrity and stability of membranes of immune cells.

Some in vitro studies have shown that short-chain fatty acids (SCFA) may exhibit immunomodulatory properties (Vinolo et al., 2011). In addition to their anti-inflammatory characteristics, SCFAs are also potent in regulating the activation and differentiation of immune cells like neutrophils, macrophages, and T-lymphocytes. Excellent sources of SCFAs are foods that are prepared through bacterial fermentation, like yogurt, cheese, pickles, soy sauce, and alcoholic beverages. Palmitoleic acid, which can be found in marine, animal, and vegetable oils, also has anti-inflammatory characteristics.

Micronutrients

Unlike macronutrients that are required by the body in large quantities, micronutrients are needed in smaller amounts. However, even though they are required by the body in smaller quantities, micronutrients play a vital role in the body, particularly in your immune system. Their deficiency can have detrimental effects on the body. Micronutrients are either in the form of vitamins or microminerals.

Vitamins

There are various vitamins that assist in boosting your immune system, both innate and adaptive. Innate immunity is immediate, while adaptive immunity is not.

Vitamin C plays a crucial role in both innate and adaptive immunity. The recommended amount for vitamin C consumption is 25–90 micrograms per day (Chaari et al., 2020). Enough consumption of vitamin C reduces oxidative damage in the body while increasing phagocytosis. It is reported that impaired immunity that is caused by vitamin C deficiency increases the severity of pneumonia, as well as other infections. Phagocytes and lymphocytes are stimulated by this vitamin.

Vitamin D is another important vitamin to your immune system. This vitamin can be obtained from a few foods. However, there are vitamin D supplements that can be of help, too. The recommended daily intake for vitamin D is 15–20 micrograms per day (Chaari et al., 2020). Vitamin D plays an important role in maintaining the integrity of mucosal cells in innate barriers, both structurally and functionally. Such innate barriers include the skin and the respiratory tract, both of which can aid viral infection if the mucosal cells are not well-maintained. Vitamin D can also enhance the differentiation process of monocytes to macrophages. Additionally, it promotes the movement of the differentiated macrophages, as well as their phagocytic abilities. Vitamin D also increases the release of inflammatory cytokines while lowering that of pro-inflammatory cytokines by macrophages. All these activities by vitamin D improve the immune system's response against infections.

You also need **vitamin B** for enhanced recovery. Vitamin B includes eight different vitamins, all of which are water-soluble. B vitamins are usually involved in cell metabolism. Grains, seeds, nuts, and liver are some of the main sources of vitamin B. Here are some of the vitamins that fall under the vitamin B category:

- **Vitamin B2**, also called riboflavin, is involved in regulating the differentiation and function of immune cells. It does so by regulating fatty acid oxidation. The recommended daily amount of vitamin B2 is between 0.6 and 1.3 milligrams each day.

- **Vitamin B3** has a central role in aerobic respiration. It is also referred to as nicotinic acid. Its role in modulating your immune system is through inhibiting the production of pro-inflammatory cytokines by monocytes and macrophages. Vitamin B3 concentration of 8-16 milligrams per day is recommended as adequate.

- **Vitamin B5**, also called pantothenic acid, is another B vitamin. Its major role is in the oxidation of fatty acids, as well as in the tricarboxylic acid (TCA) cycle. Also known as the Krebs cycle, the TCA cycle involves a series of chemical reactions that work together to release energy that is trapped in carbohydrates, proteins, and fats. In much the same way, vitamin B5 plays a crucial role in energy generation by immune cells. This role of vitamin B5 is of paramount importance to COVID-19 patients as it enhances their recovery. The amount of pantothenic acid that is regarded as adequate is 3-5 milligrams per day.

- **Vitamin B6** is a cofactor in amino acid, nucleic acid, as well as protein biosynthesis. Due to this function, vitamin B6 plays a crucial role in the synthesis of cytokines and antibodies. It is also important for the production and differentiation of immune cells.

A diet that includes vitamin B6 ranging between 0.6 and 1.7 milligrams per day is considered to be adequate for the vitamin to play its role in the body. Inadequate intake of vitamin B6 negatively impacts the proliferation and differentiation of lymphocytes, in addition to impairing the response of antibodies.

- **Vitamin B7** is a cofactor for the enzymes fatty acid synthase and acetyl-CoA carboxylase. This way, it takes part in the metabolism of fats, carbohydrates, and proteins. Also called biotin, vitamin B7 inhibits the production of pro-inflammatory cytokines. For you to benefit from the activities of vitamin B7, you should ensure that your intake of this vitamin is between 1 and 3 micrograms each day.

- **Vitamin B9**, which is also known as folate, is required by the body for protein synthesis. It, therefore, affects the production of some proteins that are part of the immune system, especially antibodies. The recommended amount for vitamin B9 is 200–400 micrograms per day. Inadequate amounts of vitamin B12 in the body reduces the production and circulation of CD8+ cytotoxic cells. This reduces the body's protection after infection while reducing the rate at which one recovers. One experimental study showed that vitamin B9 supplements increased innate immunity in elderly people (Bunout et al., 2004).

- **Vitamin B12** is mainly involved in the metabolism of carbon and folate. When your intake of vitamin B12 is below recommended concentrations, you risk having a significant reduction in the number of lymphocytes in your body. Additionally, the cells that are involved in cell-mediated immunity are greatly reduced. Inadequate amounts of vitamin B12 in your diet affect the ratio of CD8+ and CD4+ cells in the body. Some studies have also shown that deficiency of vitamin B12 lowers the response of antibodies (Maggini et al., 2007). A diet with an approximate concentration of vitamin B12 between 1.2 to 2.4 micrograms per day is considered enough for the functions of the vitamin in the body.

Microminerals

The source of most microminerals is the soil. Plants then take up these minerals and use them as part of various processes. Humans can then eat minerals by incorporating plants into their diets. Animal meat is also a source of minerals because some animals are herbivores. In this section, we will discuss different minerals and their roles in boosting your immune system.

- **Magnesium**: Your body needs a daily intake of 320-420 milligrams per day. With such an intake of magnesium, you can enhance the functioning of your immune system. Magnesium helps to regulate the activity of leukocytes. It also plays an important role in maintaining the ratio between CD8+ and CD4+ cells. Adequate amounts of magnesium also help to reduce the levels of cytokines that are involved in inflammation. Dry beans, nuts, seeds, greens, and whole wheat grains are great sources of magnesium.

- **Zinc**: The recommended daily concentration of zinc ranges between 2 and 11 milligrams per day. This important micronutrient has a key role in both innate and adaptive immunity. People with inadequate amounts of zinc have reduced numbers of immune cells, as well as the activity of those that are available. Individuals with zinc deficiency are more susceptible to infection by pathogens. The structural and functional integrity of mucosal cells is also enhanced by the presence of zinc. You can include zinc in your diet by eating dairy products, red meat, poultry, and oysters.

- **Selenium:** This macronutrient has antioxidant activity. It reduces oxidative stress that is caused by reactive oxygen species that are produced by the metabolic processes in the body. The presence of this mineral in the body has an influence on immune responses. It also reduces the production of pro-inflammatory cytokines, particularly interleukin 6 (IL-6). Some research studies have linked adequate intake of selenium with reduced severity of pneumonia-related illnesses (Chelkeba et al., 2015).

Water

Water should always be part of your diet. Drinking warm water is even better because it is regarded as an immune booster. Besides, three-quarters of your body is made up of water. Your body requires a balance of electrolytes, and this is made possible through the presence of adequate water in the body. Water also plays a crucial role in the detoxification of the body. Water is also part of your blood, so without enough water intake, it is more likely that you might reduce the amount of blood in your circulatory system. You need to drink plenty of water!

Foods That Boost the Immune System

While generally eating well has a huge impact on a stronger immune system, there are certain foods that specifically have positive effects on the immune system. When your immune system is weak, a lot of opportunistic infections can easily infect you, thereby slowing down your recovery from the effects of COVID-19. Some flu viruses can easily invade you. In this section, we are going to focus on some of the foods that you can easily get from your local grocery store. Try getting these foods, prepare them appropriately if need be, and incorporate them into your diet.

It is crucial to note that the foods that we will discuss in this section cannot prevent you from contracting COVID-19. They can only boost your immune system and enhance a quicker recovery from long COVID. Otherwise, you still have to maintain all COVID-19 regulations of social distancing, disinfecting surfaces, sanitizing hands, as well as properly washing hands with soap and running water.

1. Citrus Fruits

Citrus fruits are a good source of vitamin C, which is very good at boosting the immune system. This vitamin is reported to increase the production of white blood cells, which are an important component of the immune system. Unfortunately, the body cannot produce vitamin C on its own, so it should come from your diet. Oranges, lemons, limes, grapefruit, and tangerines are some of the good sources of vitamin C that you can grab from your grocery store. The recommended daily intake of vitamin C is 75 milligrams for women and 90 milligrams for men (National Institutes of Health, 2017). It is crucial that you note that the vitamin C from various citrus fruits can quicken your recovery from colds and cases of flu, but there is currently no evidence that shows that they can alleviate other symptoms of COVID-19.

2. Broccoli

Broccoli is one of the vegetables that are rich in vitamins and minerals. It is an excellent source of vitamin A, C, and E. These vitamins have important roles to play in enhancing the immune system. Broccoli also contains large amounts of antioxidants. These are compounds that minimize the activity of free oxidative radicals in the body. The metabolic processes that take place in the body usually release free radicals that can cause cellular damage in the body. Antioxidants remove these free radicals, thereby protecting cells, proteins, and enzymes from possible damage. Other studies have reported that antioxidants improve certain immune responses (Bendich, 1993).

You should minimize heat processing on vegetables like broccoli so that you maintain as many nutrients as possible. Heat can degrade some of the nutrients in food. Steaming is the best way to cook broccoli because it keeps the vitamins, minerals, and other antioxidants intact.

3. Garlic

Since time immemorial, garlic has been used as a traditional medicine to treat various infections. Even now, garlic is added to various concoctions and infusions that are used to alleviate symptoms such as cough. Even more importantly, garlic is one of the foods that boost the immune system. Its efficacy in doing this is aided by the presence of sulfur-containing compounds, like allicin. Some studies have reported improved immune responses from treatment with allicin, in addition to increased production of pro-inflammatory mediators (Feng et al., 2012). You can benefit from such positive effects from eating garlic and hasten your recovery from long COVID.

4. Red Bell Peppers

One of the most common assumptions that people make is that citrus fruits are the best sources of vitamin C. This is far from the truth, considering that some vegetables, such as red bell peppers, have three times as much vitamin C as that in oranges. One Florida orange provides you with about 45 milligrams of vitamin C, while one red bell pepper can give you approximately 127 milligrams (Schend, 2020). Red bell peppers are also rich in beta carotene, which has been reportedly shown to increase the number of immune cells, as well as the overall activity of the immune system.

Long sickness, as is the case with long COVID, may affect the health of the skin and eyes. The beta carotene in bell peppers can be converted into vitamin A, which is crucial for healthy skin and eyes.

5. Yogurt

Yogurts are great immune boosters, but not all of them are. Be sure to choose the ones which are labeled "live and active cultures." Such yogurts contain live bacterial cultures that may trigger your immune system into action, thereby protecting you from infections. While you recover from long COVID, you wouldn't want other infections to start attacking you and worsen your health status. Just by eating some yogurt regularly, you enhance protection.

You can even enhance your yogurt by adding some fruits to it. For unsweetened yogurts, you can add a few drops of honey. Also, select types of yogurt that are fortified with vitamin D, which regulates the immune system. Vitamin D also enhances your body's natural response against diseases.

6. Green Tea

Green tea contains a type of phenolic compound called flavonoids. This phytochemical is an antioxidant, and as we alluded to earlier, antioxidants contribute to boosting the immune system. While black teas also contain flavonoids, green tea additionally contains higher amounts of epigallocatechin gallate (EGCG), which is another antioxidant. The unavailability of EGEG in black tea is due to the fermentation process in making this tea, which destroys the EGEG. Since green tea is steamed, EGEG remains intact and available for use in enhancing the immune system (Nance et al., 2014). Green tea is also rich in L-theanine, an amino acid that is reported to enhance the production of protective compounds in T-cells. As part of the immune system, T-cells are immune cells whose responsibility is to attack specific foreign particles that invade your body. Their specificity is due to the fact that they attach foreign bodies in an antigen-specific manner.

7. Poultry Meat and Soup

Have you ever heard of the recommendation to drink some poultry soup if you are not feeling well? Well, if you have never heard about it, I have just let you know about it. Poultry, be it turkey or chicken, is rich in vitamin B6. This vitamin improves immune responses to various diseases, as well as inflammation. Vitamin B6 also contributes to various chemical reactions that occur in the body. It also plays an important role in the production of new red blood cells that transport oxygen around the body.

8. Sunflower Seeds

Did you ever think that sunflower seeds could be one of the foods that increase the efficiency of your immune system? They are because they contain a wide range of nutritional compounds, including vitamin B6, phosphorus, vitamin E, and magnesium. Phosphorus boosts the immune system. It also acts against pathogenic microorganisms that attack the body. Phosphorus also maintains a stable and healthy environment for beneficial microorganisms in the gastrointestinal tract. All these properties of phosphorus are protective to the body, hence being accounted as part of the body's immunity.

It has been demonstrated in rodents that magnesium plays an important role in cell-mediated immunity and the synthesis of immunoglobulin G (IgG) (Galland, 1988). Cell-mediated immunity is a branch of immunity that does not involve antibodies but cells such as phagocytes and lymphocytes. Vitamin E is found in significant abundance in immune cells, as compared to other cells of the body. It is an antioxidant that modulates the function of the immune system.

9. Ginger

After being sick for a long time, ginger is also one of the foods that you might need to incorporate into your diet. The efficacy in alleviating inflammation makes ginger a good food to turn to after illnesses that cause sore throat, like COVID-19. Any other forms of inflammation and nausea that result from long COVID can be addressed using ginger. Ginger can also reduce chronic pain.

## 10.	Papaya

Papaya is another great source of vitamin C, which is an immune system booster. Additionally, the fruit also contains magnesium and phosphorus, the minerals that contribute to the efficient functioning of the immune system. Folate, which is also available in papaya, is also implicated in cell-mediated immunity. Papaya also contains papain, which is an enzyme that is known for its anti-inflammatory properties.

More Nutrient Sources for Better Recovery

Nutrient	Sources
Vitamin C	Kiwi, brussels sprouts, oranges, strawberries, cabbage, cauliflower, cantaloupe, broccoli, and grapefruit.
Vitamin E	Wheat germ, hazelnuts, sunflower seeds and oil, safflower oil, peanuts and peanut butter, spinach, almonds, and tomato.
Vitamin D	Yogurt, salmon, eggs, sardines, tuna fish, cod liver oil, whole wheat grains, milk, orange juice, and mushrooms.
Zinc	Chicken, pork chop, yogurt, cashews, beef patty, lentils, beans, pumpkin seeds, and chickpeas.
Vitamin A	Carrots, red peppers, eggs, spinach, beef liver, mango, cantaloupe, sweet potato, and Ricotta cheese.
Vitamin B	Eggs, green vegetables, citrus fruits, avocados, bananas, fish, red meat, poultry, whole grains, milk, cheese, beans, and lentils.
Iron	Baked potatoes, green leafy vegetables like spinach, cereals, whole grain bread, beans, and lentils.
Selenium	Beef, chicken, fish, turkey, beans, nuts, shellfish, peas, lentils, eggs, soy products, and seeds.
Magnesium	Dark chocolate, legumes, seeds, tofu, nuts, whole grains, avocados, dry beans, wheat germ, spinach, almonds, cashews, fish, green leafy vegetables.

Chapter 6: The Cycle of Breathlessness

After COVID sickness, patients can have problems breathing well. They may experience breathlessness, sometimes. Clinically, breathlessness is denoted as dyspnea. It is usually identified through observed labored breathing and a breathing rate that is abnormal. This chapter will focus on how to manage breathlessness. Refractory breathlessness is abnormal breathing that persists, even after treatments for a certain condition or other reversible symptoms have been done. You will also learn different breathing techniques and exercises that will assist you in coping.

Tools for Monitoring Breathlessness

To begin with, we will look at different tools that are used to measure and monitor breathlessness.

Breathlessness Questionnaires

The complexity of breathlessness lies in the fact that the patient is in a better position to determine what they are feeling more than anyone else. This makes using questionnaires an important tool in monitoring the breathlessness of an individual. Using questionnaires helps health practitioners to understand the breathlessness from the patient's point of view. That way, they can make assumptions and conclusions based on the patient that they would have gotten from the horse's mouth. Questionnaires also provide the patient with a chance for self-evaluation that helps them to determine whether their condition is improving or deteriorating.

Health professionals can also create questionnaires while the patient is still acutely sick, say, in the hospital. This will help them to compare the patient's information against the observations that they make. At the end of the day, they will attain a clearer and better picture of what the patient may be experiencing.

It should, however, be noted that questionnaires require more time for them to be valid, even up to years. Moreover, they require a team of professionals to be set in place to ensure that the questionnaires cover all angles.

Various factors should be considered when selecting a questionnaire for assessing and monitoring breathlessness. Some of these factors are:

- **The patient population that was used to create the questionnaire**: There are many conditions that may cause breathlessness. Therefore, health professionals need to be sure that the questionnaire addresses the case at hand. In fact, in this case, questionnaires that are prepared using a COVID-19 patient population will be ideal and more useful.

- **The features of breathlessness are being investigated**: Breathlessness questionnaires address certain aspects of the condition. These aspects are determined by the way breathlessness affects the patient's life. For instance, breathlessness may negatively impact the overall quality of life, limited independence in carrying out activities, as well as anxiety, fear, and distress. Unfortunately, there is no questionnaire that accommodates all these aspects at once. If the aspects that need to be investigated are many, then different questionnaires are needed.

- **Is the questionnaire assessing breathlessness in relation to sedentary patients or in response to activities?** In severe cases of breathlessness, patients are usually unable to do activities. In some cases, they can do light activities. While breathlessness can be assessed in the sedentary state, it is also crucial to investigate its extent during activity.

- **What about the method through which the questionnaire is administered?**: Whichever method is used to administer the questionnaire, it should allow the patient to complete it independently. There should be no influence whatsoever. If someone has to read the questionnaire to the patient, then they have to read out the questions as they are written. The patient's answers should also be noted without alteration. From what I have explained, you might have noted that questionnaires can be administered physically or even over the telephone.

Scales for Single Item

There are scales that focus on one aspect at a time, like the visual analog scale (VAS) and Borg scale. The patient's breathlessness is measured against a scale that runs from 0 to 10. On the scales, 0 represents normal breathing, while 10 is for severe breathlessness. On the Borg scale, the numbers are used to denote the severity of the breathlessness. For instance, 2 may represent "slight breathlessness," while 7 represents a "very severe" case of breathlessness. These scales can only measure one symptom at a time. For example, you might measure "the distress that results from the breathlessness" or "the level to which the breathlessness is uncomfortable" (Yorke and Savin, 2010). To measure different symptoms using these scales, you might have to repeat the test, changing the symptom under observation each time.

The fact that the scales have numbers that represent a continuum of the patient's experience with breathlessness is thought to increase their reliability. The scoring system for these scales is not complicated, and they are easy and quick to use.

Medical Research Council (MRC) Dyspnea Scale

This scale is used to determine the different activities or tasks that trigger breathlessness. The MRC Dyspnea scale is divided into five grades, from 0 to 5. Zero denotes that one has no problems of breathlessness unless they have engaged in strenuous activities. Five represents the severe form of breathlessness, where an individual finds themselves too breathless to leave their house.

The disadvantage of the MRC Dyspnea scale is that it changes within short periods of time. However, it is a great tool for assessments that take place over longer periods of time. It can be used to check if rehabilitation procedures are leading to improvements in breathing patterns.

Transitional Dyspnea Index (TDI) and Baseline Dyspnea Index (BDI)

Both the BDI and TDI assess breathlessness in a more comprehensive way. The TDI is usually used as the initial assessment, while the TDI serves as a follow-up assessment. The BDI investigates breathlessness in three dimensions, namely, impaired functionality, how much effort, as well as how big the task is at any given time. Simply said, the BDI measures breathlessness in relation to the size of the task at hand and the effort required to complete it. The dimensions that are measured by the BDI are compared against a scale that runs from 0 to 4, with 0 representing no impairment, while 4 denotes severe breathing impairment. The TDI is then used to determine whether interventions that were done in response to the results from the BDI brought any changes. The main advantage of the BDI and TDI combination is that it can provide information on the breathing condition of the patients on a daily basis.

The Dyspnea-12

This tool helps to determine the severity of breathlessness in patients. It includes both physical and affective aspects of breathlessness. The physical element focuses on how the patient feels about their breathing. For example, they may say, "I put in too much work just to breathe." The affective component concentrates more on the emotional effects of the patient's breathing. For instance, they may say, "I am bothered by the way I breathe." After considering both the physical and affective aspects of breathing, the Dyspnea-12 tool determines the overall score. The sum of all responses is used to conclude the severity of one's breathlessness and should range between 0 and 36.

St George's Respiratory Questionnaire (SGRQ)

The SGRQ is self-administered and consists of 76 questions that the patient should respond to. Overall, the questionnaire addresses three domains, namely, symptoms, activity, as well as the effects of the condition under investigation of everyday life. Usually, breathlessness is analyzed as one of the effects on daily activities. It is also assessed as one of the symptoms, along with other symptoms such as cough, sneezing, and production of sputum. Although the SGRQ is presented in more than 100 languages as of now, it is laborious and time-consuming.

Anxiety and Breathlessness

In long COVID patients, breathlessness can be a result of the physical impact of the pandemic. However, in some cases, COVID-19 is not necessarily the direct factor for breathlessness. In such cases, the emotional effects of the pandemic may come into play. In this section, we will explore one such emotion, which is anxiety. Sometimes, anxiety can be mild. In some cases, breathlessness can be experienced by COVID-19 patients as an effect of anxiety, and this is one of the severe cases. This could be the anxiety of whether they will feel better and recover. Some become anxious about their lives with regard to whether they will survive the illness, especially considering that large numbers of people are losing their lives to it. Some begin to fear for their children, spouses, and other family members' lives. The reasons for anxiety in patients that are experiencing long COVID are countless. It is also interesting to note that breathlessness may also cause anxiety.

Here are some of the symptoms that show that you might be experiencing the anxiety that might cause breathlessness:

- Feeling nervous
- Tension in the muscles
- The feeling that danger is lurking
- Tightness in the chest
- Body weakness
- Restlessness
- Difficulty in focusing on tasks or activities

How Anxiety Affects Breathing Patterns

Your body is wired in such a way that when there is something wrong, it naturally responds in a certain way. This response is controlled by the autonomic nervous system. This system is dependent on its two branches, namely, the sympathetic and parasympathetic nervous systems. The sympathetic nervous system is the one that triggers your body to enter the "fight or flight" mode when it is under stressful conditions. In this case, your brain will be assuming that you are running for your dear life. Anxiety is one of the ways through which the body responds to conditions of stress. This response is accompanied by hormonal and physical changes such as the ones that we discussed earlier. It is the responsibility of the parasympathetic nervous system to restore the body to its original state of calmness.

Normally, when you are in calm conditions, you breathe in a much more relaxed manner. This is contrary to what you experience when you are in stressful conditions that trigger anxiety. When you're anxious, the triggers by the sympathetic nervous system increase the rate at which your adrenaline is secreted. This increases your heart rate and blood pressure. Your lung airways become wider, and this is coupled with an increase in the breathing rate. These changes can be so instantaneous to the extent that you might not even notice them. However, they happen because your mind will be assuming that your muscles require more oxygen so that you can either run or fight.

Anxiety may then lead to a state of hyperventilation. Unlike some cases where hyperventilation is a result of exhaling more air than you inhale, the one that is induced by anxiety is usually due to breathing in too much oxygen. The high amounts of inhaled oxygen are contracted by too high concentrations of exhaled carbon dioxide. Under normal circumstances, you would assume that breathing in high amounts of oxygen should make you feel just fine.

However, the fact that large amounts of carbon dioxide are equally expelled from the body makes your breathing more overwhelming than you can imagine. It would seem like you are working too hard to sustain your breathing. You might even feel like you are suffocating and as if you are not getting enough air. The following symptoms best describe the experience: confusion, dizziness, nausea, as well as a stinging sensation in your hands, lips, and feet.

Surprisingly, noticing that your breathing patterns have changed can also cause or increase anxiety. Just realizing that you are struggling to supply your lungs with enough oxygen can raise feelings of anxiety. You might even think that you are having a heart attack. Your automatic response to this could be to gasp for more air as you endeavor to take deep breaths. This would be in an effort to compensate for the inadequate supply of oxygen to the lungs. While this could possibly work, overcompensation can worsen the situation by increasing your state of anxiety, which in turn triggers breathlessness again. This becomes a cycle of breathlessness and anxiety.

Tips for Managing Anxiety-Induced Breathlessness

From the explanation that I have given, you might resonate with some of the aspects that are involved in anxiety-induced breathlessness. Even if you haven't experienced these things yet, knowing about them beforehand is an advantage. This goes along with the saying that reads, "To be forewarned is to be forearmed." Now that you understand the possibly unending cycle of breathlessness and anxiety, you should know how to stop it. For that reason, the purpose of this section is to provide you with tips that can assist you in conquering either the anxiety that causes breathlessness or the breathlessness that causes anxiety.

1. Engage the Parasympathetic Nervous System

As long as your sympathetic nervous system keeps sensing some form of danger lurking around, it will continue to operate in an effort to help your body survive the stressful situation. However, you should help your body to return to its calm state by engaging the parasympathetic nervous system. Imagine the parasympathetic nervous system as emergency brakes that help you to stop and avoid even more danger. When you engage the parasympathetic nervous system, your heart and breathing rates will subside toward normal levels. Your blood pressure will also reduce, while your muscles will relax. This way, your body returns to its calm state.

2. Use Grounding Techniques

This is a great way to relax your body and relieve anxiety in the process. Grounding techniques involve clenching and relaxing different body parts. So, basically, you should direct your entire focus on a certain part of your body, clench it and then release. You then move on to the next body part, and so on.

3. Breathe Through Your Nose

Your brain regards breathing with your mouth as a coping mechanism in times of emergencies. So, when you breathe through your mouth, your brain interprets as though you are in some form of danger and will trigger the sympathetic nervous system. Besides, when you breathe through your mouth, that's when you gasp for more oxygen than is necessary, thereby triggering hyperventilation.

You can, therefore, trigger your parasympathetic nervous system by forcing yourself to breathe through your nose. That way, your brain will interpret that the situation has normalized and will call off the alarm. In the next section, we will discuss breathing exercises that can help you to activate the parasympathetic nervous system, a step that will induce calmness.

4. Distract Yourself Mindfully

When you realize that anxiety is beginning to creep on you, you can find things that distract you from focusing on its triggers. Even the simplest distractions will do a great job. For example, you can focus on the color of the walls of your house or how beautiful the flowers in your garden are. The idea is for you to focus on something more positive while occupying your thoughts so that they are unavailable to anxiety triggers.

5. Practice Self Care

There are many self-care practices that can help you to relieve anxiety. You could write down how you feel as a way of releasing them. Whatever makes you feel better will do you great. Maybe, you would like to light some candles that have an aroma that is pleasant to you. If you are a fan of herbal teas, you can also have a cup, but be sure not to drink caffeinated ones because they might heighten your anxiety.

6. Remind Yourself of What Is Happening

From the information that has been provided earlier in this chapter, I hope you now understand how anxiety causes breathlessness. You can use this information to save yourself from other episodes of anxiety that might trigger breathlessness. Once you notice that your breathing patterns are beginning to change or have already changed, remind yourself of what is happening to you. For instance, you can loudly remind yourself that your body is trying to get more oxygen to your tissues and muscles. Tell yourself that your heart was checked by a health professional, you are fine, and you are not going to have a heart attack. You will be surprised at the extent to which this will help you to calm down.

7. Contact a Professional Therapist

The moment you find it difficult to contain an anxiety disorder, it is recommended that you engage the services of a professional therapist. These people are properly trained to teach you how to conquer anxiety. They can give recommendations that are specific to your situation, thereby providing you with maximum support.

Breathing Techniques

COVID-19 affects the lungs and your breathing abilities, sometimes leading to breathlessness even after the major symptoms of the disease have subsided. Deep breathing techniques and exercises can be of great help in enhancing better breathing patterns. Moreover, it strengthens the lungs and diaphragm after an intense illness from COVID-19. Sicknesses that affect the respiratory system can weaken the diaphragm, making it difficult for you to have long and relaxed breaths.

It is also reported that breathing exercises are a great way to clear mucus and other fluids that might be clogging the air spaces in the lungs (Whelan, 2021). This is due to the fact that deep breathing takes in oxygen deeper into the lungs. Breathing exercises can also assist you in increasing the capacity of your lungs. That way, your lungs are better able to supply the bloodstream with enough oxygen that the rest of your body requires. Another benefit of breathing exercises is that they will help you calm down and relax while you recover from long COVID.

Breathing Exercises for Inducing Calmness

Here, we will delve more into breathing exercises that specifically address the breathlessness that is caused by anxiety. These exercises are meant to trigger the parasympathetic nervous system, thereby inducing calmness. Let's get started!

Exercise 1

This exercise is meant to help you to reestablish your normal breathing patterns after a moment of breathlessness. Follow the steps outlined below for this exercise:

1. Close your mouth and breathe in through your nose, slowly. Make sure the breath is deep enough to fill your lower lungs. This should be your major focus.
2. Breathe out in a natural way. However, make sure your shoulders remain still— only your stomach should have notable movements as you inhale and exhale.
3. Repeat this type of breathing regularly throughout the day. This will assist you in making these breathing patterns more of a norm than a planned exercise.

Exercise 2

Here is an exercise that you can do when you anticipate situations that might promote anxiety. You can also perform this exercise in the face of stress and anxiety so that you can replace these with calmness.

Follow this procedure to complete the exercise:

1. With your mouth closed, inhale slowly through your nose. The air that you breathe in should initially be directed to your lower lungs before you begin to fill in your upper lungs.
2. Hold your breath while you count up to three.
3. Slowly breathe out through your mouth. Be sure to keep your stomach, face, and shoulders as relaxed as possible while you exhale.
4. Repeat this procedure over and over again.

Exercise 3

The exercise that I am going to describe now is also known as the countdown exercise. When you decide to do this exercise, make sure you have ample time to complete it properly because it takes more time compared to other breathing exercises that are meant to calm you down.

Here is how you can do the countdown exercise:

1. Find a place to sit, with your mouth and eyes closed.
2. Quietly repeat the word 'relax' while you slowly breathe in through your nose.
3. As you steadily breathe out, count down from ten until you get down to one.
4. The moment you reach one, silently tell yourself that it is time to release the tension, fear, and anxiety. Begin to imagine the anxiety departing from you.
5. Once you are convinced that the tension and anxiety have gone, open your eyes and live your new reality of calmness.

More Breathing Exercises

Although we discussed more about exercise in Chapter 4, the main focus of the simple exercises that are described in this chapter is to improve your breathing ability. You can just wake up and start walking around your room while you focus on how you are breathing. Some of the exercises that I will describe in this section are accompanied by some fun, which makes them much easier to perform.

Deep and Relaxed Alternate Breathing

Follow these steps and gradually improve your breathing techniques and ability (NHS Foundation Trust, 2020):

1. Start by breathing in a relaxed manner for about 30 seconds.
2. Make four deep breaths, followed by 30-second relaxed breathing again.
3. Repeat steps (1) and (2).
4. Huff, and then cough if necessary.
5. Repeat step (1).

You can go through all the steps of this breathing exercise as many times as you wish.

Face-Down Deep Breathing

This type of breathing targets your diaphragm. It also helps to unclog the air spaces in your lungs. Please, be sure to stop this exercise as soon as you realize that it causes difficulty breathing. Here are some steps that you can follow to perform this type of breathing:

1. Lie down on your stomach, be it on your bed, couch, or a floor with a mat. Let your hands rest on your forehead to allow for proper breathing.

2. Ensure that your mouth is closed while you keep your tongue in contact with the roof of your mouth.

3. Inhale slowly through your nose, taking the air as deep as possible. You can measure this by how deep your belly button will push itself into the mattress or whatever you are lying on.

4. Now, begin to exhale through your nose at the same rate at which you inhaled. It has to be slow.

5. Repeat the inhale-exhale exercise 10 times more.

Breathe and Hum

This breathing technique builds your ability to hold air in your lungs for longer periods of time. Here is how you can perform this breathing exercise:

1. Find a space where you can either sit or stand in an upright position. Ensure that your spinal cord is as straight as possible.

2. Place your right hand on your breastbone while you put the other one on your belly.

3. Close your mouth and ensure that your tongue touches the roof of your mouth.

4. Slowly breathe in with your nose, with your concentration fixed on pushing the

hand that is holding your belly outwards. This should be followed by the upward movement of your chest that then pushes the hand that is on your chest.

5. Slowly breathe out through your nose, but this time, accompany this step with a humming sound.

6. Repeat the breathing procedure for an average of nine times.

Yawn and Smile

This exercise is a combination of deep breathing and movements. This makes it more fun and less difficult to perform. In addition to enhancing strength due to the movements that are involved, the exercise also works on your coordination acumen. Moreover, it also helps the muscles in your chest to open up, thereby giving more room for your diaphragm to expand. Here are the steps that you can follow for this exercise:

1. Find a space where you can sit upright. This could be a chair or on the edge of a bed.

2. Lift up both arms simultaneously until they reach overhead. Yawn as you do this.

3. Bring your arms down and smile the moment they hit your laps. Maintain the smiling position for 4 seconds.

4. Repeat this procedure as many times as you can.

Pursed Lip Breathing

This type of breathing helps you to get higher concentrations of oxygen into your lungs. Moreover, it keeps the airways of your lungs open for longer since it lowers your breathing rate. This means that this type of breathing reduces the number of breaths that you take within a minute.

To try pursed lip breathing, follow this procedure:

1. Sit in an upright position, making sure that your shoulders and neck are straight but relaxed.
2. Close your mouth so that you can breathe using your nose. This is important because when you breathe through the nose, the air that you breathe in is humidified in the nasal passages before it reaches the lungs. This is impossible when you breathe through your mouth.
3. Through your nose, slowly breathe air in as you count up to five.
4. Now, you have to breathe out, but before then, purse your lips as you pretend as if you were going to blow a candle out.

5. While your mouth is still pursed, empty your lungs by breathing out slowly through your mouth. Exhale this way while you count up to eight or more.

6. Repeat steps (2) to (5) at least 10 times.

Chapter 7: Fatigue Management

It has been long predicted that COVID-19 patients are more likely to suffer from a neuroimmune condition that depletes their energy (Rockett, 2020). Due to this loss of energy, some may not be able to attend their daily job as they used to do before they were infected. Some may even become bedridden as a result. One study even reported that 50% of COVID-19 survivors experience fatigue, even 10 weeks after their initial infection (Van Beusekom, 2020). This relates to the notion that COVID-19 survivors would experience energy depletion. Fatigue is evident in most COVID patients, regardless of the severity of their experience with the COVID-19 illness.

Normally, it is recommended that people should return to their workplaces 4 weeks after viral infections. This is done to avoid deconditioning, which is a condition whereby an individual's functionality is gradually reduced as a result of prolonged episodes of inactivity. It cannot be denied, however, that fatigue related to COVID-

19 is a cause for concern, and interventions for it should be highlighted to help long-COVID patients.

It is tempting to assume that the fatigue caused by coronavirus disease is the same as what an individual feels when they are generally tired for any other reason. However, these two are not the same. While one can feel tired anytime, for any other reason, post-viral infection fatigue is experienced after a viral infection. It is not clear why post-viral fatigue occurs, but it is assumed that it is due to the cytokines that are released in response to the initial infection by the virus. It is known that one of the symptoms that result from cytokine release is tiredness. Inflammation of the nervous tissues during a viral infection can also cause post-viral fatigue.

The symptoms of post-viral fatigue are similar to those exhibited by people suffering from chronic fatigue syndrome (CFS), which is also known as myalgic encephalomyelitis. This is a condition that is characterized by long-term tiredness, accompanied by a number of other symptoms. Post-viral tiredness might be alleviated by more sleep, as compared to general tiredness. Physical and mental hard work may also increase post-viral fatigue, such as the one caused by coronavirus infection.

Here are some of the fatigue symptoms that are associated with COVID-19:

- Physical and mental tiredness
- Feeling exhausted
- Being easily agitated
- Lack of energy
- Finding it difficult to complete given or daily tasks
- Constantly feeling overwhelmed

Energy Conservation

Everything that you do is an exercise; it is just that some activities are more energy demanding than others. Energy conservation involves managing your choices concerning the tasks that you should carry out and the time that you take to complete them. As you recover from COVID, avoid beginning with more energy-demanding tasks because they might only compound your fatigue. Light tasks like making your bed are less daunting to your body. Even as you complete light tasks, you should pay close attention to your body and rest when you feel you cannot continue with the task.

Also, take note of the time frames within which you complete your tasks. A light task that is finished within a shorter period of time can require more energy than when the same task is completed within longer time frames. The whole idea of energy consumption is based on the rate at which the task is being completed. The longer the time frame, the slower the rate of completion, and the lesser the energy required to get done with the task at any given time. The opposite is also true.

Even when you have larger tasks that await your attention, break them into smaller chunks that you can manage. Perform these small tasks that together lead to the completion of the larger tasks. Be sure to rest after completing each of them to avoid overworking yourself. Another way to conserve energy is by organizing your space in such a way that the things you use most are always as close to you as possible. When your daily tools are out of reach, then there is a greater probability that you will have to move around a lot just to complete your tasks.

Plan your day and know what you intend to do during the day. This helps you to limit tasks and activities to what you can actually manage. Do not compare yourself with others because their condition is not the same as yours. Build up activities and tasks as you go, depending on how energetic you feel as days go by.

Conserving Energy in Your Daily Activities

There are things that you can decide to stop doing when you are overwhelmed with fatigue. On the other hand, there are other activities that you might not be able to run away from. They are simply part of your life, and usually, you are left with no choice but to do them. I will, therefore, highlight some tips that will help you to conserve energy, even as you do these daily activities.

Walking

Keeping the things that you need as close to you as possible helps you to minimize walking, but at some point, you will still walk. After surviving an infection with the coronavirus, walking might be a big job due to post-viral fatigue. However, you can avoid long walks, especially soon after the COVID-19 symptoms have subsided. Maybe, you can begin with shorter walks, such as going to the bathroom.

Lower Your Pace

The pace at which you do things can either relieve or worsen your fatigue. Doing things at a faster rate is likely to be more tiring than doing the same things at a much slower pace. Having said this, you should start by doing things slowly and increase your pace as you recover.

Getting Yourself out of Your Bed

When you have been bedridden for some time, getting out of your bed can be a daunting task. It can be energy-draining, but maybe you still need to get out of bed, anyway. Suppose you need to take your bath. How do you get out of bed with all the fatigue? Here is a tip: wake up slowly and sit at the edge of your bed. Rest for a little while before you can stand and go to take your bath. After taking your bath, be sure to rest again.

Climbing Up and Down the Stairs

Going up and down the stairs is another daily task that drains your energy. The best way to deal with this is to minimize the need to climb up and down the stairs. You can bring down everything that you need downstairs or rather keep them there. That way, you conserve the little energy that you have.

Getting Dressed

After taking your bath, you will need to get dressed. Make sure all the clothes that you want to wear are close to you. Remember, the goal is to conserve as much energy as you can to avoid worsening the state of fatigue. Moving around to get each piece of clothing that you want to put on can eat up your energy reserves. Also, you could consider sitting on your bed or chair while you dress. Slip-on shoes are much easier to put on, so consider wearing those if possible. This might reduce the need to bend down.

Fatigue and Your Diet

We addressed more about nutrition and diet in Chapter 5. However, this section will delve more into investigating different types of foods to determine whether they reduce or increase fatigue. As we discuss, you will notice that some of the foods that you like are probably the ones increasing your fatigue and delaying your recovery in the process.

Energizing Foods That Beat Fatigue

Food choices have been highly impacted by the increased availability and variety of foods throughout the globe. It has become more difficult than ever to determine which food is good for your health and which ones could be harmful. However, in that pool of foods, you should be able to pick the ones that serve the purpose that you want them to fulfill. In this case, we want to discuss the different types of foods that you should consider if you intend to reduce fatigue.

Fruits and Vegetables

Although all fruits and vegetables are generally considered healthy, I would recommend that you eat the seasonal, fresh ones. Mind you, what you need in fruits and vegetables are the nutrients that they contain. Fresh vegetables and fruits have higher nutrient content compared to processed ones. Fruits and vegetables that are processed would have been stripped of some of the nutrients that they contain in a bid to increase their shelf life.

Fresh fruits that you eat in their season are more likely to have ripened naturally, making them a better source of nutrients. The opposite is true for fruits that you eat when their season is over. Eat more fresh and seasonal fruits and vegetables and give yourself some energy.

Lean Meats

Meat that has a lot of fat might seem attractive to your eyes and taste buds, but it causes even more fatigue. Instead of consuming those, consider eating leaner meats like turkey, fish, and chicken, with less saturated fat. Such foods are energizing to your body.

Seeds and Nuts

Nuts and seeds are among the best energizing foods that exist. Apart from beating fatigue, these foods keep you feeling fuller for longer. If you want the best out of seeds and nuts, try to eat them raw and without salt. Sunflower seeds, walnuts, hazelnuts, pumpkin seeds, and almonds are examples of seeds and nuts that you can eat to fight against fatigue.

Unprocessed Foods

Generally, processed foods have fewer nutrients compared to the same types of foods that are not processed. As I explained earlier, foods that are processed tend to lose their nutritional value in the process, and this makes them less nourishing. The preservatives, trans fats, and other artificial ingredients that are added to processed foods will actually slow you down rather than energize you.

Whole Grains

Whole grains are a great source of nutrients incomparable to refined carbohydrate sources. This is because the refining process makes foods lose some of their nutrients. This automatically makes refined food such as white flour less energizing.

Water

We cannot conclude the discussion about energizing foods without mentioning water. Although it does not provide energy in the form of calories, water provides the medium in which metabolic processes that release energy can take place. Consider replacing soda drinks with water and make it a habit, as you will be surprised by the result. You will feel more energetic and for longer, too.

Foods to Avoid

Now you have an idea of the foods that you should consider incorporating into your diet to ensure that they help you to reduce fatigue. Exploring foods that promote fatigue is also worthwhile because it enlightens you on the types of foods that you should avoid.

Added Sugar

Added sugar is generally not recommended for any diet, and this is even more so for people who need to correct fatigue symptoms. When you eat added sugars, they are quickly broken down to glucose, thereby causing an immediate surge in energy. This energy is not long-lasting. It is quickly used up by the body, and you immediately feel tired and hungry, too.

Sugars such as fructose also cause inflammation in the body. Besides, they need nutrients for them to be processed by the body. As a result, they use up the nutrients in the body, further adding to your fatigue. I would recommend that when you have a sweet tooth, you can eat fruits because they can help you to soothe your craving and provide you with vitamins and other beneficial nutrients at the same time.

Pasta and White Rice

These are examples of refined foods that we discussed in the previous section. These foods quickly increase your blood sugar levels when you eat them, but this won't last. You will soon crash. Instead of energizing you, refined foods will suck your available energy.

Caffeine

Caffeine also triggers temporary surges in blood sugar. Moreover, it is a stimulant, so it can affect your sleeping patterns, thereby causing even more fatigue. If you just want to have the coffee flavor over your taste buds, I recommend that you stick to decaffeinated products.

Hydrogenated Oils

This is one of the most difficult foods to avoid as it is usually part of the food that people are fond of. Hydrogenated oils are found in foods like margarine, cake mixes, and candy. In addition to causing inflammation to your body, hydrogenated oils also aggravate your fatigue symptoms. Here are some strategies that you can employ to avoid some of the hidden hydrogenated oils in your favorite foods. Make it a habit to make your cakes from scratch instead of using cake mixes. Instead of eating candy bars, rather opt for dark chocolate, which even contains polyphenols that can help you alleviate fatigue symptoms.

Fried Foods

Many restaurants make money through fried foods. However, if your goal is to alleviate fatigue symptoms, you better watch out for this type of food. Fried foods are prepared by heating food in super-heated oils at high temperatures. When this happens, oxidative free radicals are produced. The moment you eat fried foods, you also take in these harmful free radicals into your body. This way, you put your body at risk of inflammation and increased fatigue. Baked and broiled foods are a better replacement for fried foods when you are eating out. At home, rather use cooking methods such as baking, roasting, and steaming.

Bananas

Many people assume that all fruits and vegetables are energizing. On the contrary, there are a few that you should avoid if you are fighting fatigue, and these include bananas. Since they are rich in potassium, bananas enhance heart health and nerve function. However, they are also rich in magnesium, which has a role to play in aiding sleep. Due to this characteristic, bananas can make you feel tired.

Alcohol

Alcohol is one of the things that you should eliminate from your diet if you are dealing with fatigue. Although alcohol might seem to be quite reviving when things are fine, the opposite could be true in an already fatigued body. Some alcohols have high sugar content, which makes them vehicles for causing fatigue. Alcohol can slow down the heart, liver, and other parts of the body, making the overall being less energetic. Making your own drinks could be the best way to avoid refined sugars embedded in some commercial drinks, particularly alcohol.

Vegetable Oils

Vegetable oils are usually regarded as "must-haves" in kitchens by many people. This is because they are used for baking, greasing pans, and frying. Since they are highly refined, vegetable oils are highly oxidized when they are heated. As a result, when you eat them, you are more likely to take in free oxidative radicals that will contribute to even more fatigue. When vegetable oils oxidize, they are converted to trans fats, which raise bad cholesterol levels in the body when consumed. Bad cholesterol can clog your arteries and deter the normal flow of blood. You can replace vegetable oils with avocado oil or coconut oil. You can consider olive oil for low-temperature cooking.

Fruit Juices

You probably considered fruit juices to be the equivalent of fruit servings. They are, but only to a certain extent. However, fruit juices that are sold in shops have a high content of added sugar, as well as preservatives and flavors. Some even have added colorants. In addition to that, even those fruit juices that are squeezed from actual fruits do not contain the fibers that are present in real fruits. That makes them less nutritious than the actual fruits. The best liquid that you can ever drink, instead of fruit juices, is water. Try it, and you will feel the refreshing characteristic of water.

Exercise for Relieving Fatigue

We discussed much more about exercises for long COVID patients in Chapter 4. Even though this time the exercise is aimed at alleviating fatigue, the rules for initiating and continuing with exercises remain the same. You still have to exercise according to the different phases of exercises that are there. You have to make sure that you can do the exercise in a lower phase with much ease before you can proceed to the next phase. Unfortunately, rushing to the exercise phase that is above your current ability may worsen your fatigue instead of relieving it.

Assuming that you now understand that you should allow for a smooth transition through phases as you try to reengage in exercises, it is important to explore how exercise may alleviate fatigue. When you exercise, the production of hormones that are called endorphins is boosted. Endorphins are also called 'happy' hormones. They can energize you while they increase concentrations of oxygen that are available in the blood at any given time.

More interestingly, an intense session of exercises can immediately make you feel even more drained, but in the long run, you will begin to feel more energetic. This is because your body is not acquainted with the level of activity that you would have engaged in at first. As you consistently exercise, it also upgrades, and that is when you begin to feel energetic. However, please keep in mind the fact that you can only undertake intense exercise sessions much later after you have gone through other exercise phases, as we discussed earlier. Regular exercise also helps to increase the quality of your sleep. This is another way through which exercises can energize you while reducing fatigue.

One study done by the University of Georgia shows that sedentary people can reduce fatigue by 65% if they engage in regular exercises of low intensity (Science News, 2008). This is quite a huge reduction in fatigue without engaging in an intense exercising session. Analysis of the results from the same study suggested that highly fatigued people can benefit more from low-intensity exercise than they would from moderate to high-intensity exercise. This was brought about by the fact that fatigued participants responded better to low-intensity exercises as compared to moderate-intensity ones. That 'little' exercise can go a long way in helping you fight fatigue.

How to Manage Fatigue

If you are experiencing fatigue after a COVID-19 infection, there are ways that you can use to manage and possibly alleviate the fatigue. In this section, we are going to focus on the different methods that you can employ in alleviating and managing fatigue.

Pain Relief Medication

Over-the-counter painkillers, like Paracetamol, can help you to alleviate some of the pain that emanates from long COVID. Pain can make you feel like the fatigue is worse and unmanageable. Therefore, relieving the pain can go a long way in making you feel better.

Monitor Your Sleeping Patterns

Generally, taking a nap helps you to feel better when you wake up. This is why it is recommended. However, you need to be careful how you do it. Sleeping for long periods of time, especially during the afternoon, may even worsen your fatigue. It is better for you to take short naps, separated by intermittent periods of being awake.

More interestingly, taking pain relief medication, as highlighted earlier, can help you to have a deeper and more peaceful sleep. This is because it is easier to fall asleep in the absence of pain than in its presence.

Train yourself to have strict sleeping patterns. You should sleep at the same time every day and wake up at relatively the same time in the mornings. You can do this by setting your alarm for the time that you should wake up. Be sure to obey the alarm when it rings because that will mark the beginning of good sleeping habits that might help you to manage fatigue.

Approach Health Professionals

When you discover that there is no noticeable improvement in your fatigue as time elapses, consider contacting a health professional for help. They can give you customized recommendations that cater to your own situation. Be sure to follow the recommendation of health professionals to the tee so that you can assess your progress.

Conclusion

COVID-19 has become a song that even kids have grown to know. However, most people assume that once the major symptoms of the disease have disappeared, then all is well within the survivors. However, this is usually not the case because there is long COVID. From reading this book, you might have been able to diagnose yourself with long COVID. Alternatively, you might have realized that someone that you know is suffering from this condition. The trauma that follows COVID-19 sickness has a negative impact on people's lives, yet it is, to some extent, underrated.

In this book, we have addressed various aspects that are related to recovery from long COVID. However, more focus is on how you can cope and manage the situation so that you can hasten your recovery. Practical ways to address some symptoms and conditions that are associated with long COVID have been provided in this book. The recommendations that have been provided in this book take a three-dimensional approach. This way, the recommendation addresses three aspects that are negatively impacted by long

COVID. These are the physical, psychological, and emotional aspects.

Psychological aspects: There are behavioral changes that help you to quicken the rate at which you recover from the symptoms of long COVID. The activities that enhance behavioral challenges, as highlighted in this book, target your mind because the root of all behaviors that you exhibit lives there. Interventions such as meditation, hypnotherapy, and applying the Law of Attraction are powerful tools in aligning your mind to the behaviors that you expect. These procedures work best when you give them space in your everyday life. For instance, practicing meditation every day makes a greater difference than doing it once in a blue moon. The same applies to the Law of Attraction. It should become more of a habit for best results.

Physical aspects: After many illnesses, getting back to doing exercise is recommended. However, with long COVID, care has to be taken to ensure that the transition from being sedentary to resuming exercise activities is smooth, gradual, and appropriate. If such care is not taken into account, the exercises might have detrimental health effects instead of enhancing healing as initially intended. There are various factors that are considered in order to determine what type of exercises a patient can engage in. The extent to which their health was negatively affected by COVID-19 is one of the major considerations. Since the severity by which people are affected by COVID-19 varies with individuals, exercise activities are categorized into phases, from 1 to 5. The difficulty, effort required, and activities increase as the phase numbers increase. This implies that phase 1 exercises require less activity compared to those in phase 5.

You should be sure of the exercises that you can do, depending on the severity of the COVID symptoms that you experienced, as well as the long COVID symptoms that you are going through. It is also important to note that you cannot juggle from, say, phase 1 exercises, to phase 4 ones. You should follow the transition smoothly between the phases to prevent shocking your body with activities that it is not ready for.

Have you ever heard of the saying "You are what you eat"? This saying implies that what you eat has a role to play in your overall being. In this case, what you eat impacts the rate at which you recover. The nutrients that food contains are what makes food so influential in determining your health conditions. The various nutrients in the food that you eat have different functions, some of which can help you recover well, especially after severe illnesses like COVID-19. In this book, different macronutrients and micronutrients have been explained, together with their roles in enhancing your immune system. The effects of various vitamins in promoting increased efficiency of the immune system have also been explored.

The reason why diet was mainly explored with reference to its effects on the immune system is that it is usually compromised, especially after illnesses such as COVID-19.

Therefore, the idea is to encourage you to eat food that boosts your immune system so that your recovery is not delayed or completely hampered. The mechanisms of action of the different nutrients in enhancing the functioning of the immune system vary. For example, some promote the proliferation and differentiation of immune cells.

Emotional aspects: It cannot be denied that long COVID has a huge impact on the emotional well-being of patients. One of the symptoms of the emotional attack that is caused by long COVID is anxiety. It is unfortunate that anxiety can cause breathlessness, which is both unpleasant and dangerous to the patient. However, this is not the end of the story. This book provides you with tips that help you to conquer anxiety and related breathlessness. Most of these tips are based on engaging the parasympathetic nervous system. For instance, you can train yourself to breathe through your nose rather than your mouth. When you breathe through your mouth, your brain decodes this as denoting a state of danger that needs an emergent response. As a result, the sympathetic nervous system triggers the fight and flight mode.

Various breathing exercises have also been recommended in order to deal with anxiety. In addition to that, breathing exercises assist you in strengthening your diaphragm and lungs. The capacity of your lungs is also improved.

I would like to congratulate you on getting to the end of this book. This is one of the best things that you have done for yourself. Now, it's time for you to create change in your life by applying the recommendations that have been made in this book.

I wish you all the best on your recovery journey, and I believe that you have been empowered, through reading this book, to experience the changes that you have always wanted to see.

For more information, please visit the following websites: www.thehealthandfitnesscoach.co.uk

or_www.thehealthandfitnesscoach.com. However, in the event that you notice unusual or worsening symptoms, be sure to contact health professionals near you for proper assistance.

References

Allen, S. (2018). *Acute respiratory distress syndrome: Causes, symptoms, and diagnosis.* Healthline. https://www.healthline.com/health/acute -respiratory-distress-syndrome

American Thoracic Society. (2020). https://www.thoracic.org/patients/patien t-resources/resources/cpet.pdf

Astuti, I., and Ysrafil. (2020). Severe Acute Respiratory Syndrome Coronavirus 2 (SARS-CoV-2): An overview of viral structure and host response. *Diabetes & Metabolic Syndrome: Clinical Research & Reviews,* *14*(4). https://doi.org/10.1016/j.dsx.2020.04.02 0

Bendich, A. (1993). Physiological role of antioxidants in the immune system. *Journal of Dairy Science, 76*(9), 2789– 2794. https://doi.org/10.3168/jds.S0022- 0302(93)77617-1

Black, R. (2015, October 6). *5 Foods to avoid if you have chronic fatigue syndrome.* everydayhealth.com. https://www.everydayhealth.com/news/fo

ods-avoid-you-have-chronic-fatigue-syndrome/

Boston University. (2020, November 19). *Three reasons why COVID-19 can cause silent hypoxia: Biomedical engineers use computer modeling to investigate low blood oxygen in COVID-19 patients.* ScienceDaily. https://www.sciencedaily.com/releases/2020/11/201119153946.htm

Branca, M. (2020, November 18). *Small study reveals details of brain damage in COVID-19 patients.* Harvard Gazette. https://news.harvard.edu/gazette/story/2020/11/small-study-reveals-details-of-brain-damage-in-covid-19-patients/

Bunout, D., Barrera, G., Hirsch, S., Gattas, V., de la Maza, M., Haschke, F., Steenhout, P., Klassen, P., Hager, C., Avendano, M., Petermann, M., & Munoz, C. (2004a). Effects of a nutritional supplement on the immune response and cytokine production in free-living Chilean elderly. *Journal of Parenteral and Enteral Nutrition, 28*(5), 348–354. https://doi.org/10.1177/0148607104028005348

Cegolon, L., Javanbakht, M., & Mastrangelo, G. (2020). Nasal disinfection for the prevention and control of COVID-19: A scoping review on potential chemopreventive agents. *International Journal of Hygiene and Environmental Health, 230,* 113605. https://doi.org/10.1016/j.ijheh.2020.1136 05

Cennimo, D. J. (2021, April 30). *How did the coronavirus outbreak start?* www.medscape.com. https://www.medscape.com/answers/250 0114-197402/how-did-the-coronavirus-outbreak-start

Centers for Disease Control and Prevention. (2019). *When and how to wash your hands.* Centers for Disease Control and Prevention. https://www.cdc.gov/handwashing/when-how-handwashing.html

Chaari, A., Bendriss, G., Zakaria, D., & McVeigh, C. (2020). Importance of dietary changes during the coronavirus pandemic: How to upgrade your immune response. *Frontiers in Public Health, 8.* https://doi.org/10.3389/fpubh.2020.004 76

Chelkeba, L., Ahmadi, A., Abdollahi, M., Najafi, A., Ghadimi, M. H., Mosaed, R., & Mojtahedzadeh, M. (2015). The effect of parenteral selenium on outcomes of mechanically ventilated patients following sepsis: a prospective randomized clinical trial. *Annals of Intensive Care, 5*(1).

https://doi.org/10.1186/s13613-015-0071-y

Cherry, K. (2019). *How meditation impacts your mind and body.* Verywell Mind. https://www.verywellmind.com/what-is-meditation-2795927

Coronavirus recovery: Breathing exercises. (n.d.). www.hopkinsmedicine.org. Retrieved May 15, 2021, from https://www.hopkinsmedicine.org/health/conditions-and-diseases/coronavirus/coronavirus-recovery-breathing-exercises

Cronkleton, E. (2019, April 9). *10 Breathing exercises to try: For stress, training and lung capacity.* Healthline. https://www.healthline.com/health/breathing-exercise

Davis, N. (2018, September 17). *You can do this low-impact cardio workout in 20 minutes.* Healthline. https://www.healthline.com/health/fitness-exercise/low-impact-cardio

Elmer, J. (2018, August 15). *Shortness of breath and anxiety: Symptoms, causes, and treatment.* Healthline. https://www.healthline.com/health/shortness-of-breath-anxiety

Esser, N., Legrand-Poels, S., Piette, J., Scheen, A. J., & Paquot, N. (2014). Inflammation as a link between obesity, metabolic syndrome and type 2 diabetes. *Diabetes Research and Clinical Practice, 105*(2), 141–150. https://doi.org/10.1016/j.diabres.2014.04.006

Everlywell. (n.d.). *COVID-19 and nutrition: Care for yourself and others with these tips: Home health testing made easy - Results you can understand.* www.everlywell.com. https://www.everlywell.com/blog/covid-19/covid-19-and-nutrition/

Fatigue after COVID-19. (n.d.). www2.Hse.ie. https://www2.hse.ie/conditions/coronavirus/fatigue-after-coronavirus.html

Fehr, A. R., & Perlman, S. (2015). Coronaviruses: An overview of their replication and pathogenesis. *Coronaviruses, 1282*, 1–23. https://doi.org/10.1007/978-1-4939-2438-7_1

Feng, Y., Zhu, X., Wang, Q., Jiang, Y., Shang, H., Cui, L., & Cao, Y. (2012). Allicin enhances host pro-inflammatory immune responses and protects against acute murine malaria infection. *Malaria Journal, 11*(1), 268. https://doi.org/10.1186/1475-2875-11-268

Fraley, L. (2020, June 5). *Coronavirus and shortness of breath: What does it feel like?* Healthline.

https://www.healthline.com/health/coron
avirus-shortness-of-breath

Galland, L. (1988). Magnesium and immune function: An overview. *Magnesium, 7*(5-6), 290–299. https://pubmed.ncbi.nlm.nih.gov/307524 5/

Garg, S. (2020). Hospitalization rates and characteristics of patients hospitalized with laboratory-confirmed coronavirus disease 2019 — COVID-NET, 14 States, March 1–30, 2020. *MMWR. Morbidity and Mortality Weekly Report, 69.* https://doi.org/10.15585/mmwr.mm6915 e3

Giovinco, J. (2020, June 9). *"It feels like you're drowning with no water:" Survivor says damage done by COVID-19 may follow him for life.* FOX 13 News. https://www.fox13news.com/news/it-feels-like-youre-drowning-with-no-water-survivor-says-damage-done-by-covid-19-may-follow-him-for-life

Goldberg, E. L., Molony, R. D., Kudo, E., Sidorov, S., Kong, Y., Dixit, V. D., & Iwasaki, A. (2019). Ketogenic diet activates protective γδ T cell responses against influenza virus infection. *Science Immunology, 4*(41), eaav2026. https://doi.org/10.1126/sciimmunol.aav2 026

Grant, M. C., Geoghegan, L., Arbyn, M., Mohammed, Z., McGuinness, L., Clarke, E. L., & Wade, R. G. (2020). The prevalence of symptoms in 24,410 adults infected by the novel coronavirus (SARS-CoV-2; COVID-19): A systematic review and meta-analysis of 148 studies from 9 countries. *PLOS ONE*, *15*(6), e0234765. https://doi.org/10.1371/journal.pone.023 4765

Groth, L. (2020, April 30). *Muscle pain is a symptom of COVID-19—Here's how it feels.* Health.com. https://www.health.com/condition/infecti ous-diseases/coronavirus/is-muscle-pain-a-symptomarotene-of-coronavirus

Han, C., Duan, C., Zhang, S., Spiegel, B., Shi, H., Wang, W., Zhang, L., Lin, R., Liu, J., Ding, Z., & Hou, X. (2020). Digestive symptoms in COVID-19 patients with mild disease severity. *American Journal of Gastroenterology*, *115*(6), 916–923. https://doi.org/10.14309/ajg.000000000 0000664

Hanes, E. (2021, April 19). *Breathing exercises to help long-term COVID effects.* Healthgrades. https://www.healthgrades.com/right-care/coronavirus/breathing-exercises-to-help-long-term-covid-effects

Headspace. (2019). *What is meditation?* Headspace. https://www.headspace.com/meditation-101/what-is-meditation

Headspace. (2020). *What are all the types of meditation and which one is best?* Headspace. https://www.headspace.com/meditation/techniques

Healio. (2018). *Components of the immune system.* Healio.com. https://www.healio.com/hematology-oncology/learn-immuno-oncology/the-immune-system/components-of-the-immune-system

Holland, K. (2017, January 25). *Is my blood oxygen level normal?* Healthline. https://www.healthline.com/health/normal-blood-oxygen-level

Jewell, T. (2021, March 2). *2019 coronavirus (COVID-19): Symptoms, treatment, prevention.* Healthline. https://www.healthline.com/health/coronavirus-covid-19

Jiang, B., & Wei, H. (2020). *Oxygenation and ventilation.* COVID-19 Treatment Guidelines. https://www.covid19treatmentguidelines.nih.gov/critical-care/oxygenation-and-ventilation/

Kaiser Permanente. (n.d.). *Beta-carotene.* Wa.kaiserpermanente.org. https://wa.kaiserpermanente.org/kbase/topic.jhtml?docId=hn-2804006

Kay, L. (2020, June 13). *Why COVID-19 makes people lose their sense of smell.* Scientific American. https://www.scientificamerican.com/article/why-covid-19-makes-people-lose-their-sense-of-smell1/

Khanna, R., Cicinelli, M., Gilbert, S., Honavar, S., & Murthy, G. V. (2020). COVID-19 pandemic: Lessons learned and future directions. *Indian Journal of Ophthalmology, 68*(5), 703. https://doi.org/10.4103/ijo.ijo_843_20

Kim, G. U., Kim, M. J., Ra, S. H., Lee, J., Bae, S., Jung, J., & Kim, S. H. (2020). Clinical characteristics of asymptomatic and symptomatic patients with mild COVID-19. *Clinical Microbiology and Infection.* https://doi.org/10.1016/j.cmi.2020.04.040

Klopfenstein, T., Kadiane-Oussou, N. J., Toko, L., Royer, P.-Y. ., Lepiller, Q., Gendrin, V., & Zayet, S. (2020). Features of anosmia in COVID-19. *Médecine et Maladies Infectieuses.* https://doi.org/10.1016/j.medmal.2020.04.006

Krans, B. (2015, March 23). *Foods that beat fatigue.* Healthline. https://www.healthline.com/health/food-nutrition/foods-that-beat-fatigue

Lewis, E. D., Meydani, S. N., & Wu, D. (2018). Regulatory role of vitamin E in the immune system and inflammation. *IUBMB Life, 71*(4), 487–494. https://doi.org/10.1002/iub.1976

Li, P., Yin, Y.-L., Li, D., Woo Kim, S., & Wu, G. (2007). Amino acids and immune function. *British Journal of Nutrition, 98*(02), 237. https://doi.org/10.1017/s0007114507699 36x

Lima, C. M. A. de O. (2020). Informações sobre o novo coronavírus (COVID-19). *Radiologia Brasileira, 53*(2), V–VI. https://doi.org/10.1590/0100-3984.2020.53.2e1

Lindberg, S. (2018, September 28). *RPE: What does this scale tell you about exercise?* Healthline. https://www.healthline.com/health/RPE

Long Covid Support. (n.d.). *Log into Facebook.* Facebook. https://web.facebook.com/LongCovidPag e?_rdc=1&_rdr

Maggini, S., Wintergerst, E. S., Beveridge, S., & Hornig, D. H. (2007). Selected vitamins and trace elements support immune function by strengthening epithelial barriers and cellular and humoral immune responses. *British Journal of Nutrition, 98*(S1), S29–S35. https://doi.org/10.1017/s00071145078329 71

Maragakis, L. (2020, June 25). *Coronavirus and COVID-19: Who is at higher risk?* www.hopkinsmedicine.org. https://www.hopkinsmedicine.org/health/conditions-and-diseases/coronavirus/coronavirus-and-covid19-who-is-at-higher-risk

Mathur, B. (2020, September 16). *Food rich in protein, micronutrients and hydration are key in COVID-19 recovery, say experts.* NDTV-Dettol Banega Swasth Swachh India. https://swachhindia.ndtv.com/national-nutrition-month-coronavirus-food-rich-in-protein-other-micronutrients-and-hydration-are-central-in-covid-19-recovery-say-experts-50092/

Mayo Clinic. (2020, August 21). *COVID-19: Who's at higher risk?* Mayo Clinic. https://www.mayoclinic.org/diseases-conditions/coronavirus/in-depth/coronavirus-who-is-at-risk/art-20483301

Miedaner, T. (2015, February 25). *3 Laws of Attraction: Starting with the present is always perfect*. LifeCoach.com. https://www.lifecoach.com/articles/laws-of-attraction/3-laws-attraction-the-present-is-always-perfect/

Miller, A. (2020, November 10). *What you need to know about post-viral fatigue*. Patient.info. https://patient.info/news-and-features/what-you-need-to-know-about-post-viral-fatigue

Moore, S. (2015, September 7). *How positive thinking really can change your life*. Greatist. https://greatist.com/connect/law-of-attraction

Mozes, A. (2021, February 4). *Study: Young COVID survivors can get reinfected*. WebMD. https://www.webmd.com/lung/news/20210204/study-young-covid-survivors-can-get-reinfected

Mukamal, R. (2020, May 22). *Eye care during the coronavirus pandemic*. American Academy of Ophthalmology. https://www.aao.org/eye-health/tips-prevention/coronavirus-covid19-eye-infection-pinkeye

Nance, C. L., Mata, M., McMullen, A., McMaster, S., & Shearer, W. T. (2014). Regulation Of innate immune recognition of viral infection by Epigallocatechin Gallate. *Journal of Allergy and Clinical Immunology,* *133*(2), AB246. https://doi.org/10.1016/j.jaci.2013.12.876

National Foundation for Infectious Diseases. (2020, January 25). *Coronaviruses.* National Foundation for Infectious Diseases. https://www.nfid.org/infectious-diseases/coronaviruses/

National Institute on Aging. (2016). 15-minute sample workout for older adults from Go4Life . *YouTube.* https://www.youtube.com/watch?v=Ev6y E55kYGw

National Institutes of Health. (2017). *Office of dietary supplements - Vitamin C.* Nih.gov. https://ods.od.nih.gov/factsheets/Vitamin C-Consumer/

National Institute of Allergy and Infectious Diseases. (2020). *Coronaviruses | NIH: National Institute of Allergy and Infectious Diseases.* www.niaid.nih.gov. https://www.niaid.nih.gov/diseases-conditions/coronaviruses

NHS Foundation Trust. (2020). *Covid-19 (Coronavirus) — Rehabilitation guide.* https://www.sfhtr.nhs.uk/media/8996/pil202006-01-cv19rg-covid-19-rehabilitation-guide.pdf

Nutrition and Diet. (2020, December 1). *How protein bolsters COVID-19 recovery.* www.ift.org. https://www.ift.org/news-and-publications/food-technology-magazine/issues/2020/december/columns/nutrition-and-diet-how-protein-bolsters-covid-19-recovery

O'Connell, K. (2012a, August 5). *Everything you need to know about fever.* Healthline. https://www.healthline.com/health/fever

O'Connell, K. (2012b, September 10). *Causes of fatigue and how to manage it.* Healthline; Healthline Media. https://www.healthline.com/health/fatigue

O'Neill, M. (2020, October 15). *Is a stuffy nose a symptom of COVID? Here's what an expert says.* Health.com. https://www.health.com/condition/infectious-diseases/coronavirus/is-stuffy-nose-a-symptom-of-covid

Oh, J., & Klivans, L. (2020, May 5). *How the coronavirus attacks your lungs.* KQED. https://www.kqed.org/science/1963200/how-covid-19-attacks-your-lungs

Patrick, D. R., Findon, G., and Miller, T. E. (1997). Residual moisture determines the level of touch-contact-associated bacterial transfer following hand washing. *Epidemiology and Infection, 119*(3), 319–325. https://doi.org/10.1017/s0950268897008261

Powers, K. A., & Dhamoon, A. S. (2019, April 6). *Physiology, pulmonary, ventilation and perfusion.* The National Center for Biotechnology Information; StatPearls Publishing. https://www.ncbi.nlm.nih.gov/books/NBK539907/

Public Health England. (2016, July 18). *Health matters: getting every adult active every day.* GOV.UK. https://www.gov.uk/government/publications/health-matters-getting-every-adult-active-every-day

Rockett, D. (2020, July 21). *COVID-19 patients could be at risk for chronic fatigue syndrome: "Your whole life can change if you get this."* Medicalxpress.com. https://medicalxpress.com/news/2020-07-covid-patients-chronic-fatigue-syndrome.html

Sakay, Y. N. (2020, September 1). *How does COVID-19 typically progress? A timeline for the majority of cases.* Daily Sabah. https://www.dailysabah.com/life/health/how-does-covid-19-typically-progress-a-timeline-for-majority-of-cases

Salman, D., Vishnubala, D., Feuvre, P. L., Beaney, T., Korgaonkar, J., Majeed, A., & McGregor, A. H. (2021). Returning to physical activity after covid-19. *BMJ*, *372*. https://doi.org/10.1136/bmj.m4721

Samaranayake, L. P., Fakhruddin, K. S., & Panduwawala, C. (2020). Sudden onset, acute loss of taste and smell in coronavirus disease 2019 (COVID-19): A systematic review. *Acta Odontologica Scandinavica*, *78*(6), 467–473. https://doi.org/10.1080/00016357.2020.1787505

Sanders, L. (2020, September 14). *Treatments that target the coronavirus in the nose might help prevent COVID-19*. Science News. https://www.sciencenews.org/article/coronavirus-covid-19-treatments-target-nose-prevention

Schend, J. (2020, April 30). *What to eat and drink to boost your immune system*. Healthline. https://www.healthline.com/health/food-nutrition/foods-that-boost-the-immune-system

Schoeman, D., & Fielding, B. C. (2019). Coronavirus envelope protein: Current knowledge. *Virology Journal*, *16*(1). https://doi.org/10.1186/s12985-019-1182-0

Science News. (2008, March 2). *Low-intensity exercise reduces fatigue symptoms by 65 percent, study finds.* ScienceDaily. https://www.sciencedaily.com/releases/2008/02/080228112008.htm

Scott, E. (2020, November 18). *Let the Law of Attraction help you with positive change.* Verywell Mind. https://www.verywellmind.com/understanding-and-using-the-law-of-attraction-3144808

Seladi-Schulman, J. (2019, March 29). *Post-viral cough: Symptoms, causes, treatment, and Recovery Time.* Healthline. https://www.healthline.com/health/post-viral-cough

Seladi-Schulman, J. (2020a, August 6). *Is a headache a sign of coronavirus? Is it a common symptom?* Healthline. https://www.healthline.com/health/is-headache-a-sign-of-coronavirus

Seladi-Schulman, J. (2020b, October 12). *Coronavirus loss of taste, loss of smell: Is it a common symptom?* Healthline. https://www.healthline.com/health/coronavirus-loss-of-taste-loss-of-smell#an-early-symptom

Simmons, G., Zmora, P., Gierer, S., Heurich, A., & Pöhlmann, S. (2013). Proteolytic activation of the SARS-coronavirus spike protein: Cutting enzymes at the cutting edge of antiviral research. *Antiviral Research, 100*(3), 605–614. https://doi.org/10.1016/j.antiviral.2013.09.028

Skin rash should be considered as a fourth key sign of COVID-19. (2020, September 14). Covid.joinzoe.com. https://covid.joinzoe.com/us-post/skin-rash-covid

Smith, M. W. (2020, September 23). *Your eyes and coronavirus (COVID-19).* WebMD. https://www.webmd.com/eye-health/covid-19-and-your-eyes

Staff Writer. (2018, June 25). *6 anxiety breathing symptoms and how to stop them.* Real Life Counseling. https://reallifecounseling.us/anxiety-breathing-symptoms/

Su, L., Ma, X., Yu, H., Zhang, Z., Bian, P., Han, Y., Sun, J., Liu, Y., Yang, C., Geng, J., Zhang, Z., & Gai, Z. (2020). The different clinical characteristics of coronavirus disease cases between children and their families in China – the character of children with COVID-19. *Emerging Microbes & Infections, 9*(1), 707–713. https://doi.org/10.1080/22221751.2020.1744483

Therabody. (n.d.). *5 exercises to increase athlete coordination.* PowerDot.com. https://www.powerdot.com/blogs/training/increase-athlete-coordination

Tian, Y., Rong, L., Nian, W., and He, Y. (2020). Review article: gastrointestinal features in COVID-19 and the possibility of faecal transmission. *Alimentary Pharmacology & Therapeutics, 51*(9), 843–851. https://doi.org/10.1111/apt.15731

Van Beusekom, M. 2020. (2020, November 11). *Half of recovered COVID-19 patients report lingering fatigue.* CIDRAP. https://www.cidrap.umn.edu/news-perspective/2020/11/half-recovered-covid-19-patients-report-lingering-fatigue

Vandergriendt, C. (2020, March 31). *Coronavirus types and which type is wreaking havoc worldwide.* Healthline. https://www.healthline.com/health/coronavirus-types

Varga, Z., Flammer, A. J., Steiger, P., Haberecker, M., Andermatt, R., Zinkernagel, A., Mehra, M. R., Scholkmann, F., Schüpbach, R., Ruschitzka, F., & Moch, H. (2020). Electron microscopy of SARS-CoV-2: a challenging task – Authors' reply. *The Lancet, 395*(10238), e100. https://doi.org/10.1016/S0140-6736(20)31185-5

Vinolo, M. A. R., Rodrigues, H. G., Nachbar, R. T., & Curi, R. (2011). Regulation of inflammation by short chain fatty acids. *Nutrients, 3*(10), 858–876. https://doi.org/10.3390/nu3100858

Wadman, M., Couzin-Frankel, J., Kaiser, J., & Matacic, C. (2020, April 17). *How does coronavirus kill? Clinicians trace a ferocious rampage through the body, from brain to toes.* https://www.sciencemag.org/news/2020/04/how-does-coronavirus-kill-clinicians-trace-ferocious-rampage-through-body-brain-toes

Waehner, P. (2020, April 3). *Try these 8 relaxing stretches for your entire body.* Verywell Fit. https://www.verywellfit.com/relaxing-total-body-stretches-1231150

WebMD. (n.d.). *Coronavirus and pneumonia.* WebMD. https://www.webmd.com/lung/covid-and-pneumonia

WebMD. (2019, February). *EMDR: Eye Movement Desensitization and Reprocessing.* WebMD. https://www.webmd.com/mental-health/emdr-what-is-it

Wong, C. (2003, December 11). *Mindfulness meditation.* Verywell Mind.

https://www.verywellmind.com/mindfuln
ess-meditation-88369

World Health Organization. (2020a, February).
*Report of the WHO-China joint mission
on Coronavirus Disease 2019 (COVID-19).*
https://www.who.int/docs/default-
source/coronaviruse/who-china-joint-
mission-on-covid-19-final-report.pdf

World Health Organization. (2020b, June 17).
*Criteria for releasing COVID-19 patients
from isolation.* Www.who.int.
https://www.who.int/news-
room/commentaries/detail/criteria-for-
releasing-covid-19-patients-from-isolation

WorldOMeter. (2020). *Coronavirus death toll
update - Worldometer.* worldometers.info.
https://www.worldometers.info/coronavir
us/coronavirus-death-toll/

Wypych, T. P., Marsland, B. J., & Ubags, N. D. J.
(2017). The Impact of diet on immunity
and respiratory diseases. *Annals of the
American Thoracic Society,
14*(Supplement_5), S339–S347.
https://doi.org/10.1513/annalsats.201703
-255aw

Yan, C. H., Faraji, F., Prajapati, D. P., Ostrander,
B. T., & DeConde, A. S. (2020).
Self-reported olfactory loss associated with
outpatient clinical courses in Covid-19.
International Forum of Allergy &

Rhinology.
https://doi.org/10.1002/alr.22592

Yetman, D. (2020a, April 29). *Coronavirus: Diarrhea and other confirmed gastrointestinal symptoms.* Healthline. https://www.healthline.com/health/coronavirus-diarrhea

Yetman, D. (2020b, June 4). *Is pink eye a symptom of COVID-19?* Healthline. https://www.healthline.com/health/coronavirus-pink-eye

Yorke, J., & Savin, C. (2010, April 30). *Evaluating tools that can be used to measure and manage breathlessness in chronic disease.* Nursing Times. https://www.nursingtimes.net/clinical-archive/respiratory-clinical-archive/evaluating-tools-that-can-be-used-to-measure-and-manage-breathlessness-in-chronic-disease-30-04-2010/

Yoshii, K., Hosomi, K., Sawane, K., & Kunisawa, J. (2019). Metabolism of dietary and microbial vitamin B family in the regulation of host immunity. *Frontiers in Nutrition, 6.* https://doi.org/10.3389/fnut.2019.00048

www.ingramcontent.com/pod-product-compliance
Lightning Source LLC
Chambersburg PA
CBHW051053050726
47592CB00002B/514